SUCCESSFUL AGING FOR WOMEN OVER 50

CREATE YOUR NEXT STEPS WITH CONFIDENCE AND LONGEVITY BY LIVING A HEALTHIER LIFESTYLE WITH A BODY YOU'LL LOVE!

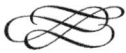

JANINE HUNKA

© **Copyright 2023 - All rights reserved.**

The content contained within this book may not be reproduced, duplicated or transmitted without direct written permission from the author or the publisher.

Under no circumstances will any blame or legal responsibility be held against the publisher, or author, for any damages, reparation, or monetary loss due to the information contained within this book, either directly or indirectly.

Legal Notice:

This book is copyright protected. It is only for personal use. You cannot amend, distribute, sell, use, quote or paraphrase any part, or the content within this book, without the consent of the author or publisher.

Disclaimer Notice:

Please note the information contained within this document is for educational and entertainment purposes only. All effort has been executed to present accurate, up to date, reliable, complete information. No warranties of any kind are declared or implied. Readers acknowledge that the author is not engaged in the rendering of legal, financial, medical or professional advice. The content within this book has been derived from various sources. Please consult a licensed professional before attempting any techniques outlined in this book.

By reading this document, the reader agrees that under no circumstances is the author responsible for any losses, direct or indirect, that are incurred as a result of the use of the information contained within this document, including, but not limited to, errors, omissions, or inaccuracies.

CONTENTS

Introduction   7

1. Taking a Step Back in Time   13
2. Stepping Into Healthy Aging From the Inside Out   37
3. Stepping Into Your Authentic Self   61
4. Step Up and Love Yourself   81
5. Stepping Into Physical and Social Activities   99
6. Step Into a Stronger Immune System   113
7. Step Into Your Power!   129

Conclusion   141
References   145

To Diane, Leann, Missy, Sue and Zella
Throughout the years whenever life got complicated and scary, I always found strength in your friendships. I've learned there's a unique and special bond I call sisterhood.

In Memory of my Mentor, my Guide, my Friend

"The Best Secret I've ever learned about life is to always find joy in every circumstance. Even in some of my darkest days, I could always find something to laugh about in the situation to restore my joy. Laughter is so good for your soul while joy remains your superpower. Always keep your head up... You got this!"
Tony Scott

INTRODUCTION

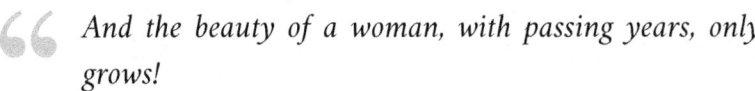 *And the beauty of a woman, with passing years, only grows!*

— AUDREY HEPBURN

It was 3 weeks before I would turn 56. I wasn't planning a massive event, merely to meet a couple of friends at my favorite restaurant for dinner and drinks. I remember waiting in the front entrance frantically texting a couple of the invitees who didn't respond yet because I knew I needed to be surrounded by as many people as possible on that day. After a certain age, birthdays just become dates to remind me that it's time to take stock of my life. Sadly, this is a venture in which I often come up short, as there are always those things I wished I did or even regretted doing, dreams I never pursued, and opportunities I allowed to slip through my fingers.

Until a few years ago, I was still married and had someone else to blame if these supposedly joyous occasions weren't as great as I had hoped. After trying to hold it all together, I think we just got so tired of pretending everything was fine and we both caved, calling our lawyers. This was the start of a 12 month battle that seemed like an eternity! When it was finally all over, the life I had for 20-odd years was amputated. This left me feeling a sense of loss, and thinking back, I had already felt a deep feeling of being lost long before signing the final paperwork.

Frankly, I didn't care anymore. I instinctively knew that the best part of my life was over, and I didn't have much hope that the years ahead would be any better. This was one idea I had absolute clarity on as it was the predominant thought consuming my mind night after night while I was lying awake, staring at the ceiling. What kept me awake? Quite simply, pain and discomfort. I was faced with many deep probing questions —whether I was a good fit to spearhead my team into the new direction the company was taking, how long it would still be until someone discovered that I wasn't the right person for the position, or even if I was financially secure enough to look after myself from now on. If it wasn't for the sheer emotional pain from this self-doubt I was feeling, I was also experiencing unexplained physical pain in my abdomen.

This pain started as sensitivity in my belly, which grew in severity and was sometimes unbearable. However, after several visits to my doctor, I still had no answers. I finally got some answers only after I was admitted for further tests.

After waiting for two weeks of painful dread, anxiety, and many sleepless nights, I was finally called in to hear the truth about my situation. This was a truth I knew would hurt me because I had to see the surgeon in person. I remember the cold, sterile waiting room where I was sitting—another number waiting to be called—with my fingers pressing into the skin of my palms as I desperately tried to anchor myself in a whirlwind of emotions.

"I'll need to operate very soon as I'm concerned the cancer may have spread. At the moment, it can still be contained in your colon. Do you have anyone to talk to about this, and do you know who can take care of you afterward?... Janine?"

"I'm sure I'll figure all that out, doctor!" were the words with which I acknowledged that my entire world came tumbling down, crashing right onto my shoulders. Of course, I'll have someone at home. I don't know who, but I'll get someone to help me. It won't be a sister, a mother, or even a child, as one might expect from someone my age, but I'll have someone. Just like that, it didn't matter whether people RSVP for any events I was planning, for I'll be in long-term recovery. It didn't matter anymore that I was divorced, for this thing happening to me was mine alone to carry.

Surgery to remove colon cancer, followed by two more major surgeries less than a year later, should've been enough to break my spirit—a spirit already fragile to begin with—but it didn't. Today, I realize that the moment I experienced in the doctor's office correlates with how most mature women are perceived in society; at that moment, with my fingers clenched into my skin, I had reached the pinnacle of that reflection. Yet, by grace alone, that moment didn't initiate a rapid decline into the deep dark valley of mature living until death—no, it was the final ledge I had to overcome to find sufficient support to propel me forward.

I am now healthy, confident, active, and happy almost a decade later. I have been challenged so much in the last 10 years than in the nearly 56 years leading up to that moment.

I am very proud of my motorbike skills. After recovering from my major surgeries, I became a much more carefree person than I've ever been before. For the longest time, I thought the right thing to do was stay within the lines while coloring all the pictures in my life. Yet, I suddenly started to find it exhilarating and fun to go over those lines and expand my horizons. By doing so, I've met so many people who share their hunger for life, a hunger that's so contagious that it got me to first learn how to ride a bike, and then I had to purchase my very own.

I reached a point where I wanted to figure out how I could add meaning to my life by helping others—I am still a volunteer and derive a great deal of pleasure from it—but I also wanted to know how I could add value to my life, simply by doing things for myself, discovering myself, making the most of my time, and taking up the interests I've always kept hidden away.

In the middle of what many would call a "midlife crisis," a medical crisis—a severe threat to my life—pulled me right back into life, a life fuller and radiant with much more wisdom thanks to maturity and experience. Reaching this low point in my life saved me as it forced me to make changes by seeking spiritual strength, living healthier, and being happier. The techniques I share in this book won't stop you from aging since nobody escapes the natural course of life. What we do have a choice over is how we age. Since we are on the mature side of the spectrum, we also have the wisdom to determine what we can control and what we can't while making the most of those things we have control over.

I've studied and read a lot about aging successfully and how to make the golden years of your life truly golden. This is an ongoing venture, and I'm still learning new things after all these years. One term that I truly found inspiring is to become a Super-ager. *Super-agers* are people on the more mature side of the spectrum but still live a life of mental and physical vitality in their 70s and 80s (Harvard University, 2017). Super-agers are often fitter, happier, and more content with the quality of their lives, finances, health, and relationships. It's the word that best describes my life now, the one I wake up to every morning after having a healthy, restful night's sleep. This life I'm living, roaming the peaks of what life has to offer after making several changes, is one most people would call a typical midlife crisis.

It's the life I wish for you and every other woman who is still super at heart, has so much to offer, and has an abundance of freedom to experience new things.

In this book, I share my story and the techniques I follow to transform my life. These techniques certainly aren't fairy tales, but are backed by science and research. These techniques help you transition into an inspired, motivated, healthy, and prosperous life. The type of life that makes life worth living and old age nothing but a mere number ensuring discounts at certain stores. It's also the type of life that serves as testimony that midlife is not a crisis but a time to celebrate. Is this the kind of life you've been hoping for?

Then dive right in!

TAKING A STEP BACK IN TIME

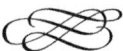

> *Aging is an extraordinary process where you become the person you always should have been.*
>
> — DAVID BOWIE

When I was about 12 years old, my friends and I would refer to our parents as "old." To us, they were old, but we also saw them in a different light. We thought of them as people who had their ducks in a row, who knew where they were heading in life, or who had already arrived at that place and were now merely waiting for us to grow up and leave the house so they could grow old in peace.

These "old" people were only in their late 30s or even approaching their early 40s. By the time I turned 38, I was still looking for my destination, and whether I would even arrive there remained questionable. Today, I know you can be in your

30s, 40s, or even your 70s or 80s and still need to get your ducks in a row.

Age is no cure for being human. Yet, through the cumulation of years, we attain a new level of wisdom. This wisdom stems from experience, regret, repeating the same cycles, and ultimately learning that some things that appeared to be such important matters are not as important as we thought. This realization often leaves me wondering why I spent so much time trying to accomplish certain goals when I can now see they're only fleeting moments in a much larger time frame.

Most of my realizations regarding aging are impacted by events that took place in the past 30 years, leaving me curious about how my life perspectives would change if I look back on this day 30 years from now. The desire to avoid repeating the same mistakes I've made until this point in my life turned into a need to know what those in their 90s regretted, appreciated, feared, and felt.

What becomes your most meaningful thoughts when you pass the 80s or 90s mark?

MAKING PEACE WITH YOUR PAST LIFE

Being human results in most people having to make peace with certain choices or actions of their past. It also means that you may need to make peace with specific past versions of how you presented yourself to the world that wasn't always a reflection of your true self.

Carl Jung introduced the world to the concepts of an authentic self and a shadow self. The renowned psychologist defined the *shadow self* as the dark side of our existence compared to the *authentic self*, which is far more enlightened and the part you want to show the world. The shadow self is where sexual drive, the desire for more power, and emotions like anger and jealousy are nestled. This idea is also echoed in the work of Erik Erikson and Donald Winnicott. All these experts in psychology determined that there are two parts to human existence—the side we show to the world and the side we keep hidden away, often necessary for survival.

Our awareness of the different sides of our personalities often begins during our teenage years, and as we explore our identity further, the matter only grows in magnitude, often leaving an even greater sense of discomfort about who we've become and the stark contrast it presents to whom we want to be. The unawareness of what is causing this internal discomfort is only amplified by the emotions we experience. As long as we don't know what's wrong, there's nothing we can do about the problems we're facing. The lack of understanding of what causes us to feel a certain way may cause anxiety. When I didn't know what was wrong with me, I would lie awake many nights dreading the worst possible outcomes. While the final prognosis wasn't a favorable one, it did give me a starting point where to begin to address my concerns. It was only then that improvement and healing could begin.

Becoming aware of the two sets of identities may not be something you like to hear as it confirms that there are dreams, goals, and hopes you may never realize. But once awareness of the situation becomes real, you can start to address that—like everyone else—you have a part of your being that will never be lived. Then you can begin to make peace with the idea. This kind of peace brings comfort in our older years because comfort comes from peace. And peace can also spark creativity, encouraging new growth and plans for the future regardless of how long it may take. Thus, making peace with the life we never lived sets us free to make the most of the time we have left, and there's no way to substitute this kind of peace that results from this revelation. Can you identify the parts of your life you'll never live? Are you ready to make peace with it?

OPPORTUNITY FOR GROWTH, NOT CRISIS

Far too quickly, the time of life which should be the most significant period of growth is labeled as a "midlife crisis." There's nothing resembling a crisis at this stage of life, and I want to explain why I oppose this conventional statement. I've stated in the previous point that making peace with these parts of our lives can spark creativity. This creativity is ultimately the soil in which new growth shoots roots.

First, I want to state that the term "midlife crisis" dates back to 1965 (Haslam, 2019). This was when Elliot James published a paper using the words for the first time in a public forum. Decades have now passed. These were decades known for exceptional progress and growth. The world back then resembles very little of what we consider the norm today. One of the areas where advancement took place was in the medical field, ensuring a longer life expectancy. And, the age that was typically considered to be midlife is no longer relevant.

Yet, within the changing world, you need to consider making changes at some point in your life. These changes will result in your internal realization that there might be more to life than you initially anticipated. You are at an age where you may have greater freedom than before. The origin of this freedom can also be based on greater financial stability, increased wisdom, and life experience. You may be in a much more favorable position now to realize dreams you once had when you were 18, 28 or even 48. The obstacles you were facing at that time may no longer be relevant.

Any situation can also look vastly different at any point in time. You may find yourself in a situation or position where you thought you might remain comfortable for years to come, only to realize changes in your environment suddenly made your situation irrelevant, or perhaps something changed so dramatically that you were no longer the best fit for that position. Then, the world you considered your comfort zone opted to push you out.

Either way, while midlife may not be a crisis, it does beg for changes to be made. Also, you might just be one of the many people in this age group that has now expanded to include everyone in the 43–62 age range—and perhaps even

onwards—who aren't prepared to shift gears to ensure a far more promising future.

This widespread unpreparedness can be due to several existing myths regarding this time. The first myth is, of course, that reaching this age is an indication that from now on, life is a downhill journey characterized by decline. It's a historically outdated assumption, as many success stories counter this understanding. Let's look at several vastly successful individuals who only had their first taste of success during their older years.

Harland Sanders, the Colonel of Kentucky Fried Chicken, franchised the brand when he was 62. Laura Ingalls Wilder, the author of the *Little House* series, started to write these books when she was 65. At an even much more mature age of 93, Harry Bernstein, the author of *The Invisible Wall: A Love Story That Broke Barriers*, started writing his book and only gained his successful reputation by the age of 96. Julia Child became a celebrity chef when she was 51, and Charles Darwin published *On the Origin of Species* when he was 50 (*Success Over 50*, 2021). These are just some of the familiar names of people whose lives speak of the opposite of decline.

There's another myth to keep an eye on; midlife is a time when magical transformations take place. The risk of this myth is that it presents this age as a time when change happens automatically and easily. It presumes that you've gathered so much life experience and learned all the lessons life had to present to you that now you can sit back and enjoy the transition without applying willpower or effort. It's not true! Change is never an easy or a comfortable process, regardless of your age. Change never happens instantly. Even if you step out today and immediately apply every technique or skill I share in this book and think change will be an easy or painless process, it will equate to falling into the trap of an illusion. Change is a gradual process, and only by consistently following the techniques and skills shared in this book, will it become a manageable venture.

By not allowing yourself to believe in these myths, you'll approach this time and use it to make much-needed changes to ensure a happy and lasting future in an entirely functional manner.

Another noticeable change that often becomes a matter of urgency during this stage is a career change. This can be a daunting obstacle to overcome, and yet this, too, can become completely manageable. First, it will demand that you open your mind to many more possibilities that are available now than what was the case when you entered the workforce for the very first time. Compared to two or maybe even three decades ago, there are far more opportunities to utilize your expertise in your field and to have the flexibility of becoming a consultant for organizations around the world. This will allow you to be more flexible timewise, charge higher fees typically linked with consultation work, and will enable you to work past the traditional retirement threshold.

You will need to cultivate an awareness of your capabilities—even those you have no formal education for but still gained experience in—and how you can apply them in a new and advanced manner in your favor. While it's relatively safe to say that most corporations aren't taking care of internal preparation and that, at some point, senior management will leave the firm to start the second part of their journey, this may be the reality you need to adjust to. It's no longer a time when retirement means sitting back and waiting to die. No, retirement is merely a beginning to a specific era of your life and the start of a brand new venture. How well you manage this transition will depend on your approach to these changes.

BANISHING REGRET

Oh, how much agony do we put ourselves through over what we should've done, could've done, or never should've done in the first place? These thoughts, from which nothing good ever comes, can keep us up all night long. And when you're carrying the burden of regret and never think about letting go of things in your past, it becomes very challenging to soar and reach your dreams.

Let's be honest—it's likely impossible to continue living a life that started out as being young and ignorant about the reality of our choices, going through many turbulent times, and having made no mistakes. The mistakes we've made are the lessons we've learned, and that's how they helped shape the people we are now. When I think about the regrets I've had over my life—and believe me, there are many—I find comfort in the words of Theodore Roosevelt in his very famous speech, *The Man in the Arena*, especially when he says (Roosevelt, n.d.): "The credit belongs to the man—or woman—who is actually in the arena, whose face is marred by dust and sweat and blood; who strives valiantly; who errs, who comes short again and again; who spends themselves in a worthy cause; who at best knows in the end, the triumph of high achievement, and who at the worst, if they fail, at least they fail while daring greatly, so their place shall never be with those cold and timid souls who neither knows victory nor defeat." (para. 1)

Reading this, I want you to ask yourself, *should I be proud of my mistakes?* Not for erring in the first place but because mistakes are yet another testimony of a life lived fully regardless of what the challenges were.

Nonetheless, regrets can be sneaky, and it's best to develop a method to banish them entirely because these regrets can develop into depression and a range of other health concerns (Adams, 2012). A great starting point is to identify the things you regret; perhaps it's a career never pursued, education never fulfilled, or an adventure you never took. Regardless of what it is, it would help if you determined the cause of any past regret. Then you can divide these into two groups: (a) the ones you need to accept, as you have no control over the situation, and (b) the ones you're still able to change. The latter leaves you with many inspiring thoughts to add to your to-do list. These things can add a new purpose to your life as you think and plan creatively about how you can realize these dreams at any age. At times, your ability to realize these dreams becomes even more significant due to your age rather than in spite of it.

The following approach is inspired by Erik Erikson's theory of *ego integrity versus despair*. It boils down to the idea that through the wisdom of maturity, you gain a greater understanding of the emotional fluctuations and challenges you've experienced during your younger years and have earned a greater sense of acceptance of your mistakes. The bottom line is you need to become kinder to yourself and stop the mental castigation over human error. Accept that there were certain things you had to do to get by, and even though you would do things much differently now, you're no longer the same person as the one who took those regretful actions. This acceptance can translate into wisdom and life experiences.

Life and the journey that took you to your present life is rarely, if ever, straightforward. There are many ups and downs, and sometimes life can appear like finding your way through a complex maze. Yet, think about all the wisdom you've gathered through these mistakes and how the knowledge you've earned can help someone else, once you begin to share it.

Once, when I had a similar conversation with another attendee at a workshop I attended, she stated that she agreed with me, but one thing still bothered her. Her cause for concern was the number of mistakes she made; according to her, there were far too many. This perspective quickly spins out of control to the point where you start to equate your value to the number of mistakes you've made. It's a message that can be further supported through past toxic relationships or even similar relationships you haven't let go of yet. Start by amputating toxic people or relationships that keep you trapped in this kind of thinking that's nothing but bondage over you. The second step is to remind yourself daily, if necessary, that your value as a person who has impacted the lives of others—often in ways you'll never know— far exceeds the value of your mistakes. You're always worth more than your mistakes, so stop beating yourself up! You're only human, and you have to find your way through life—a journey that isn't easy for most of us.

FORGIVE YOURSELF

Closely tied to the previous point is forgiving yourself. Are you familiar with that warm sensation filling you from within as gratitude flows over you once you're forgiven? Forgiveness is a gift that you should consider giving to yourself. It's the best gift you can give yourself when you want to start from a clean slate at the start of a new year, life stage, or even after a challenging circumstance.

Through forgiveness, you can come clean with yourself and the world too, as it means you are unburdening yourself to never pick up the same baggage again. It's also the best antidote to keep regret from poisoning your mind and your physical health.

"Yes, but I've already let go of past regrets," I hear you say. Sure, but have you forgiven yourself for the heartache, the destruction, or the broken relationships that your actions might have caused? Have you truly forgiven yourself as you would wholeheartedly forgive someone you love? Forgiving yourself doesn't equate to forgetting what you've done. It means you no longer punish yourself for being human and making the mistakes the rest of the world makes. It's also a vital step to enjoying a far better life.

POSITIVE THINKING

The more mature we become, the more significant the contribution of positive thinking is to our overall mental, physical, and emotional wellness. Replacing negative thoughts consuming your mind with positive alternatives can add years to your life-literally! During a 2019 study, researchers determined that positive thinking alone can contribute to more than a 10% increase in lifespan, improving the odds of living beyond 85 years (Stibich, 2020).

It also makes sense that those who are more positively inclined in their approach to life generally look forward to aging. They don't consider it as the time in their lives when every part of their existence is experiencing a steep downward decline. They look forward to the experience, regardless of what challenges this may bring, as positivity is also closely linked to greater resiliency in facing life changes or even the discomfort of illness.

One of the contributing factors to increased positivity as we grow older, which you should consider, is the greater insight that age brings. Sure, there was a time when you might have felt as if you had the world at your feet and all your skin and body parts were still firm and wrinkle-free, but this was a very shallow type of empowerment. Now you have wisdom and experience on your side, which lends itself to presenting deeper insights into the many problems which kept you confused during your younger years. These insights should also provide a deeper appreciation for your health and how to properly care for your body.

How Can You Become More Positive?

There are several habits you can include in your daily routine to help you become more positive:

- **Use a gratitude journal to recount the positives in your life**. By capturing your thoughts of gratitude in words, you amplify the value they bring to your life. Keeping such a journal can be a straightforward routine requiring little time and effort. Pick your favorite time of day and set a few minutes aside to write down the things you're truly grateful for at the moment, during the past year, or in any specific situation. Don't just scribble them down without putting any thought into it. Instead, visualize these positive memories and feel the sense of gratitude physically manifesting inside as you express authentic gratitude for what's happening in your life.
- **Use positive affirmations to transform your underlying feelings**. By repeating specific positive messages to yourself daily, you cause a gradual shift from leaning toward negative thinking and always expecting the worst to being more positive in general. A typical positive affirmation example is, "I'm feeling stronger every day." What would your positive affirmations be? Why not write them down now?
- **Use loving-kindness meditation to show yourself self-love**. This particular form of meditation is widely encouraged to increase compassion towards others and improve your ability to be kinder to yourself. I'll expand more on this later on.
- **Choose who you surround yourself with**. You've probably already realized that we become like the people we surround ourselves with most of the time. So choose wisely who you pick for the company you want

to keep. The more you spend time with people who are naturally more positive than negative, the more you'll become like them.

Does Being Positive Become Harder as You Age?

If you have been a positive person all your life, it will be easier to remain positive when you reach your midlife and beyond too. However, if you've always been the person who sees the cup as half empty rather than half full, then it may be more challenging. Is this referring to you? In that case, the following points are even more important for you, as positivity will have an even more integral role to fulfill in your life:

1. The first step to take on this quest is to remind yourself that change can happen at any time in your life. The past still remains the best time to make changes to ensure a better life, but the second best time is right now, regardless of how old you are. It's never too late!
2. Next, determine where you'll start to initiate change. There are certain aspects of your life where you have no control, and then there are many areas where you do have control and can instigate change. Identify one such area and start working on it right away.
3. Your happiness doesn't only impact your life but can also leave a positive imprint on the world. While happiness is mainly identified with being lighthearted, it's serious business because by finding your happiness, you can improve the lives of many others too.

4. Whenever you have to make a choice, choose joy! Always deliberately lean into being happier by seeking the silver lining around the dark cloud, and take every action needed to make a positive mindset part of your being.
5. I will be discussing the role of mindfulness in your life later on in this book, but for now, if you employ greater awareness and stay present in the moment, you can do wonders for your level of positivity too.

One of the biggest obstacles to enjoying a positive approach to life is the regret we feel about past mistakes. An effective way to overcome this is by dissecting the situation you regret to determine what life lessons you've learned from those moments. Examining how you've applied these lessons during other moments in your life will give you more favorable outcomes. You can then move from the perspective of looking at a life you regret to being grateful for the many ways that life has enriched your being.

CONSIDER LIFE REVIEW THERAPY

Life review therapy is based on the theory of Dr. Robert Butler, who stated that by reviewing your life and reminiscing on certain moments can bring peace and even a sense of greater control as you're more empowered over your life. Dr. Butler recommends this therapy for older adults (Nall, 2018).

This type of therapy can take on several forms and usually centers around a specific area in your life, whether it be your education, health, the music you've listened to at various times, or even the values you hold dear at certain times. While it can be a trip down memory lane, relying on specific tools to help you settle into this journey, like old photos, letters, notes, or even music, can be very beneficial.

Life review therapy can heal and help you feel calmer about the past. It can also aid in perceiving your memories and experiences from a different perspective. For example, people who suffered abuse as children often remember those horrific times from the perspective of being a scared child. Through life review therapy, you can look at the events from an adult perspective and feel greater empathy for the younger version of you who endured this abuse without the emotional maturity you have now. This can help ease the emotions you might still struggle to resolve.

Furthermore, it's also informational and can shed light on certain events that led to specific outcomes you might have forgotten about. Lastly, it's educational as you get to know yourself better.

This is a helpful aid for those who suffer from mental concerns like dementia, depression, Alzheimer's, or anxiety; people who have a terminal diagnosis; or those who have recently lost a loved one. This therapy offers hope and gives meaning to life when it may be hard to find anything positive to hold onto. It also serves as a supportive treatment to address some of the mentioned states and does wonders for self-esteem by reminding you of what you've achieved in your life.

This therapy focuses on positive events and will also help you overcome negative thinking. As a result, it serves as a way to ease the symptoms of depression. Life review therapy also increases acceptance and self-worth (Promises Behavioral Health, 2012).

While this is a recommended method to increase the level of positivity in older adults, reflection should be part of your life regardless of your age. You can make the necessary changes by reflecting on your past to improve your future.

How to Practice Life Review Therapy

① It's important to plan this type of therapy when you have enough time to sit down and review your life. Consider several 30 to 60 minute sessions spread across several days. This therapy requires a more structured approach than just sitting and remembering your life. The following steps will guide you along the way:

> ⓐ Select a specific time frame you want to reflect on. You may want to do this annually to reflect on the past year's events, or you may want to look back at your entire life for the first time. It doesn't matter when. Just have some clarity on the specific period.

② Identify certain moments or highlights in this phase that you want to review. These can be any significant moments that left a lasting impression on you. For example, during the past year, you experienced a breakup, which was devastating, but you also enjoyed recognition for the excellent work your business is doing in the community—something you're very proud of.

> ⓐ Remember that the moments leaving a lasting impression on you can seem insignificant. But to you, they may be emotionally potent, leaving a lasting impression. Therefore, when you list the moments that come to mind, remember that no moment is never too big or too small to review, and consider every possible success, failure, lesson, repeating theme, and lesson you've learned.
> ⓑ When your list is completed, arrange them into the order you want to start reflecting on. Fortunately, you have complete autonomy over what you want to reflect on and when.

③ Next, it's time to reflect. You can ask many questions to give your time of reflection deeper meaning, and I've divided them into specific groups.

> ⓐ When reflecting on success and growth, may it be personally or professionally, consider these questions:
>
>> i. What were your most significant accomplishments during this timeframe?
>> ii. What goals did you reach?
>> iii. What are some of the healthy habits you included in your routine?
>> iv. What risks did you take and are now enjoying the rewards?

v. What sort of skills did you develop during this time?

ⓑ When reflecting on your relationships and the people you surround yourself with, consider the following:

i. Who are you truly grateful for in your life?
ii. What makes specific relationships meaningful to you?
iii. What do you enjoy about any new relationships, bonds, or networks you've included in your life?

ⓒ Asking the following questions will help you to reflect on any shortcomings:

i. What was your biggest failure?
ii. List three lessons you've learned from this failure.
iii. What bad habits can you identify that you need to replace?
iv. When did you invest time or money without seeing any returns?
v. What are the goals you still need to achieve?
vi. What were the obstacles you didn't overcome?

ⓓ Use and expand on these questions to reflect on lessons or recurring themes:

i. Which events, people, or situations keep showing up in your life?
ii. What can you learn from these happenings?

iii. What lessons did you learn from the highlights you've identified?
iv. How will your past mistakes guide you to where you need to improve?
v. When capturing the period in one headline, what would it be?

④ What have you learned from these situations that constitute growth?

This exercise can take several sessions to complete.

1. Define your current reality. When you take a road trip, you have to know where you are, where you want to go, and how to get there. The same is true for your future. Defining your current position will help you determine where you want to go in life. Assess all areas individually by determining your feelings about your current financial state, health, relationships, or spirituality.
2. Plan your future. Where are you heading? What would you like to improve in your current reality? What steps do you need to take, and how can you accomplish this?
3. Once you've put your thoughts into writing, you'll enjoy greater clarity and confidence in the present moment and have much more hope for your future.

LET'S GET PRACTICAL

I grew up with the saying that "talk is cheap." It also goes along with the saying "put your money where your mouth is." So, rather than just reading how you can age gracefully and successfully, I want you to get more involved.

First, get a gratitude journal. I love stationery, so I turn journal shopping into a wonderful event. Invest in a book you would like to write in and even get a pen that sits comfortably in your hand. Decide what time of day suits you best to put a few minutes aside devoted to gratitude and capture your thoughts and feelings in your journal.

You will need more time in the second exercise, which will give you an excellent return on your investment. It's now time for a life review session. Follow the practices explained above, and always capture your thoughts and feelings in your gratitude journal too. The following questions and prompts will guide you along the way:

- When and where were you born? What were the circumstances you were born into?
- Describe your childhood years. Where did you spend most of your childhood? What was the community like? What were your parents like?
- Describe your family, siblings, and any extended family.
- What were you like as a child? What games did you like? Who was your best friend? Why?
- Detail what your teenage years were like.

- Did you study? What? When? Where? What was student life like for you?
- Did you get married? Describe the romance you've had with your partner. How did you meet? Expand on the proposal and the wedding day.
- Do you have children? Expand on their births and lives and what impact parenting has on you.
- What were the best moments as a parent?
- Did you meet any influential people?
- How many long-term friendships do you have? How often do you still have contact?
- Who were the people who had a significant impact on your life, and whose life did you impact significantly?
- What are your current living and work situations?
- Are you healthy? How active are you? What activities do you like?
- Did you experience any world-changing events? What were they like?
- How do you feel about your future? Why?

Of course, you can come up with more questions, but these will give you a great head start.

A FINAL WORD

- For some, aging is a curse, while others approach getting older with positivity and gratitude. The cause of this difference in perspective is often based on how you look at your past.

- You'll find life far more enjoyable and you'll have more hope for the future when you make peace with your past.
- You can see midlife and beyond as a crisis or a time for change to prepare for your future.
- It's easy to get hung up on regrets, and guilt will suffocate your joy; instead, banish all regrets and guilt from your life.
- Letting go of guilt and regrets are the first steps to forgiving yourself.
- People who think positively live longer—replace negative thinking with positive thinking.
- Life review therapy can change your perspective on the past and give you confidence in your future.
- As you age, one factor that has an immense impact on how you perceive your future is the state of your health. Next, we'll explore how to have successful aging through healthy living.

STEPPING INTO HEALTHY AGING FROM THE INSIDE OUT

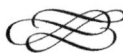

> *It takes a long time to become young.*
>
> — PABLO PICASSO

It's so easy to blame the state of our lives, emotions, or moods on others. How often do you use statements like the following?:

- "If only my husband would listen when I talk, I would be much happier with my marriage."
- "My parents divorce caused my marriage to fail."
- "Nobody can be happy working for a boss like mine."
- "I would be happy too if I didn't have all these aches and pains."
- "You know, it's my kids who cause all my sleepless nights."

If you allow outside factors to impact your internal happiness and joy, you will always be unhappy; this was one of the hardest lessons I learned. I always thought I was taking responsibility for my own happiness, but that was just a lie I told myself. If I did, then the people, things, and circumstances of my life wouldn't have impacted me for all these years. If you seek authentic and lasting joy and contentment, you need to take the journey within.

THE BENEFITS OF AGING

Aging has such a bad rap in broader society because we get so fixated on all the cons while completely forgetting about the perks of growing older.

I want to share two benefits of aging with you. There are a lot more, and I know you'll be able to think about them simply by letting your mind go in that direction. Still, these two benefits are so profound and overshadow so many other aspects of your life that I decided to only focus on these two as a foundation for your continued search for aging benefits.

As we age, something unique happens. We experience a U-curve in our happiness. Research studies indicated that from your youth to your 40s, happiness gradually declines (Rock, 2018). The outcome is that you likely experienced discomfort and discontent in your 40s. It's easy to think that you've wasted most of your life, and from this point onwards, you should expect nothing but a decline.

That is not the case, says economists David Blanchflower and Andrew Oswald. They determined in 2008 that experiencing a U-curve in your happiness is normal. This curve indicates that in countries where people have a reasonable standard of living, happiness declines until it reaches a low point around the age of 50. Then it increases again to a peak around age 70 (Rock, 2018). The appearance of this curve is described as a gradual disappearance of the shadows lingering over you. It's a time when it becomes easier to focus on internal happiness because you start to appreciate minor things and value relationships more.

I'm not saying your life will take an immense turn towards being better than what you are experiencing right now, but by looking at your life differently, in a manner fused with gratitude, it will become much more manageable. Everything in life is what you make of it. This probably isn't a new concept to you, but by applying this practice, your life will become easier and more manageable.

There's a valid reason behind this benefit of aging. This change is caused by your brain entering a new developmental stage after age 50 (Rock, 2018). While it's widely accepted that a mental decline can be expected after this age, this is untrue. Specific symptoms, like struggling to remember names, may be linked to failing mental capacities, but far too much attention is given to this. The fact that there are also positive changes taking place is usually disregarded.

Research from the Seattle Longitudinal Study determined that there's a decline in memory and speed, but due to *neuroplasticity*

—the brain's ability to change—the more mature brains are showing an increase in capabilities of spatial and abstract reasoning, verbal skills, and simple math (Phillips, 2011).

Some other changes noticed and linked to these changes in the brain after the age of 50 is enjoying a greater sense of calm. Also, if you tend to be on the neurotic side, this too will improve with age.

So don't believe everything you're told. Just because the broader assumption is that mental skills and abilities decline at a mature age doesn't mean there aren't any positive neurological changes taking place, causing you to become naturally happier after the age of 50. These changes and knowing that your brain still has more potential should inspire you to take care of your mental health and continue to challenge yourself to optimize all your possibilities.

PURPOSE IN MIDLIFE

When I think about midlife and beyond, I often have the following vision in my mind. Say you're traveling at 60 miles per hour. You don't feel that you're traveling at this speed, and there's no difference between sitting in a vehicle moving at this speed versus sitting on your couch. That is, of course, until you come to an unplanned stop. Then, if you weren't wearing your seatbelt, your body continues to move at 60 miles per hour, and you'll feel the difference when you injure yourself from the impact. For most of your life, you might have been traveling through life at a fast pace to keep up with all your responsibilities. Then suddenly you reach an age where your children don't need you anymore—you may retire, or any other significant life change may occur, leaving you free from the many things you had to take care of. Now your life moves at such a slowed-down pace compared to what you were used to that it may feel like it came to an unplanned stop. If you weren't prepared for this, the emotional impact might leave you feeling like you've traveled without a seatbelt. You may not go through a windscreen or cause yourself a severe physical injury, but it may feel like your life has no purpose.

When you still have a purpose in life, you will likely be healthier and fitter, feel better emotionally and enjoy higher levels of motivation and inspiration. Without purpose, the decline in all aspects of your life will show up much faster. A sense of purpose increases cognitive abilities and even adds to longevity.

How do you prepare for this stop and make sure your life still has a purpose after 50, 60, or any other age when life severely slows you down?

There are always significant needs in the world, and offering your services as a volunteer for a cause you feel passionate about is only one of several ways to ensure you still have a sense of purpose regardless of your age. Other tips are to learn a new skill, pick up a hobby, engage more socially, get involved in your community, or even start tutoring or mentoring younger minds eager to learn from your experience. It doesn't matter what type of purpose you pursue, but rather that you do so.

MINDFULNESS

Living mindfully and with greater awareness of the current moment you're in is beneficial during any stage of life and becomes more vital as a contributing factor to your overall wellness and longevity as you age.

The best way to describe *mindfulness* is as a consistent awareness of your emotions, experiences, thoughts, and the environment you're in. This awareness is merely an experience and not judgmental at all. Thus, you're more aware of how matters are, how you experience them and don't judge them as good or bad. Mindfulness is often linked to meditation. You can practice mindfulness in several ways, even when you're having a meal or taking a shower. Those who are more mindful tend to be calmer and enjoy a greater sense of peace in their life.

Mindfulness Benefits for Older Adults

Here are some of the benefits linked to being mindful:

- You will experience a greater sense of calm and feel more relaxed.
- This increased sense of tranquility will provide better sleep patterns.
- Lower blood pressure is another common benefit.
- Mindfulness is also a way to encourage a higher level of activity.
- It improves memory.

- It's a tool that assists you through challenges and helps you make significant transitions in life—often part of being an older adult.
- It's a coping mechanism to deal with challenging situations like chronic pain, illness, or loss.
- Mindfulness contributes to longevity and quality of life.

As these benefits become even more valuable for any older adult, aging mindfully should be something you explore daily to improve the quality of your life.

Practicing Mindfulness

The easiest way to become more mindful is to start practicing it right now. Start by setting a few minutes aside every day to slow down the pace of your thoughts and become aware of what's happening and what you're experiencing at that moment.

Let's do a quick exercise right now (Chilangwa, 2021):

1. Take a couple of deep breaths and notice what you're feeling on the outside and within.
2. Notice your thoughts, emotions, any external sensations like the sun on your back, a breeze on your face, any sounds you hear, scents you smell, or pain or discomfort you feel.
3. Don't judge any of these things—just observe them while knowing there's no right or wrong judgment,

fear, or threat. In other words, nothing is good or bad—it just is.

Start to change your way of thinking about concerns you have. Rather than fearing them from happening, accept them as part of life.

When matters upset you, identify whether there's anything you can change about the situation or whether it's beyond your control. If issues are insignificant, let them go.

You can also practice mindfulness by taking greater control over how you eat, sleep, spend your time, and how active you are.

Mindfulness can be practiced during conversations and while being social; instead of drifting off mid-conversation or thinking more about how you're going to answer, truly listen to others when they speak and notice their facial expressions and body language.

Whenever you feel overwhelmed, take a moment to pause and breathe deeply. As you shift focus from your concerns, you'll feel stress and anxiety leave your body.

Can you see how easy it is to become more mindful and enjoy mindfulness's many benefits?

Most of what I have described so far falls under the category of mindful awareness, which is one of four ways to increase your mindfulness level. The others are:

- **Mindful intentionality:** Rather than going through life on autopilot, moving from one habitual task to another, start to do things with intention. An example of this would be changing your showering or bathing approach. Instead of considering it a daily task, immerse yourself in the process and notice the warm water, the sensation of the soap suds on your skin, and the scents you smell. Be aware of how good it is to clean yourself daily and what a refreshing experience it is.
- **Mindful presence:** Stop moving from one place to the next without purpose or taking note of your surroundings; instead, become aware of your surroundings. When you shop for groceries, smell the fruit and vegetables, notice the other people, and pay attention to the sounds you hear. Even when sitting in your home, tune into your surroundings.
- **Mindful gratitude:** Gratitude plays such a vital role in your overall wellness. Use greater awareness of all the privileges you have. Instead of focusing on the fact that you would like to have a bigger home, try being grateful for the home you have; many others don't even have that in their lives. Be thankful for being able to see, hear, smell, walk, or anything else you may take for granted in your life.

MINDFULNESS MEDITATION

Mindfulness meditation is another helpful way to become more aware.

Mindfulness meditation is a form of meditation that enables you to enjoy a greater appreciation of every aspect of your being through greater awareness of the present moment without holding any judgment. While this type of meditation has its roots in Buddhist practice, it has since evolved to become a helpful tool in improving life without having to attach any spiritual meaning to it.

You may be no stranger to meditation and are familiar with the positive contribution it can make in your life. If you're not, there's always time to start. Due to the many benefits that meditation can bring to midlife and beyond, there's no better time than now to explore this practice.

Mindfulness meditation helped me move away from a place where my mind was consumed with stress over my physical health and it helped me accept my diagnosis. I was better equipped to handle the treatment and operations I had. I believe you can only truly understand the power of meditation —specifically mindful meditation—when you can visualize the benefits in your life. Some of the benefits you can expect to enjoy are feeling less stressed and anxious, reduced symptoms of depression, improved overall mental health, and a better mood in general (*Mindfulness for Older Adults*, n.d.).

PHYSICAL BENEFITS OF MINDFULNESS MEDITATION

Mindfulness meditation can improve the physical structure of your brain due to its impact on your gray matter. Changes to brain structure due to the combination of neuroplasticity and mindfulness meditation were confirmed in a 2011 study that relied on MRIs, indicating an increase in cortical thickness. This area of the brain is linked to learning and memory. At the same time, it also shows a reduction in the size of the amygdala —the brain's center for stress, fear, and anxiety (Rosales, 2018).

Improved Heart Health

Claims that meditation can improve blood pressure, insulin resistance, stress response, and heart health were proven during a study conducted by the American Heart Association in 2017 (Rosales, 2018).

Meditation Can Reduce Pain

More than 11% of the U.S. population suffers from chronic pain, and most rely heavily on prescription painkillers. It's important to be aware that this kind of medication can produce many side effects. Since studies indicate that mindfulness meditation reduces pain, I strongly recommend you try meditation to help manage your pain levels more effectively (Rosales, 2018).

Longevity and Cognitive Health

It's usually after reaching a more mature age that we're confronted with mortality. Then, like never before, we start to ponder longevity and how to enjoy a long, full, and healthy life.

Here too, mindfulness meditation comes onto the stage like a hero. Numerous studies provide sufficient scientific findings indicating that meditation improves cognitive health by reducing the impact of aging on our brains. It's said that from our mid-20s onwards, brain deterioration slowly begins, while it only shows the toll it took at a more mature age. As mindfulness meditation improves cerebral health, it slows the impact of cognitive deterioration and improves mental health, especially in the more mature section of our brain (Rosales, 2018).

Even if you're still deciding whether meditation is suitable for you, the benefits you can enjoy from meditation and mindfulness far outweigh the cost, which is essentially nothing but a minor time investment.

EMOTIONAL BENEFITS OF MINDFULNESS MEDITATION

Even though I've already covered many of the emotional benefits you can expect to enjoy when meditating regularly, the following three benefits continue to stand out:

- It increases your ability to focus and maintain your level of attention.

- You'll enjoy increased compassion for others but also be kinder towards yourself.
- Applying a greater sense of self-control becomes easier.

MINDFUL DIET

The more mature you become, the more critical it is to be aware of what you eat and how it impacts your body. Mature people who eat mindfully live longer and healthier lives because they provide their bodies with all they need, leaving them feeling healthy, focused, energized, and overall feeling better.

One of the most common reasons more mature people don't take such great care of their diet is that they find it troublesome to prepare a balanced and healthy meal for only one person or want to eat the same things when they were much younger and more active. This doesn't have to be the case, as cooking and eating are wonderful ways to socialize. Why not share healthy meals, recipes, and stories with others? Turning mealtimes into a social venture can benefit you greatly. And doing this can help you overcome specific lifestyle changes like depression and loneliness, mourning a loved one, or the feeling of rejection caused by divorce (Robinson & Segal, 2023). By turning eating times into a social event, you can even overcome the restraints of a limited budget on the food you can afford.

A mindful diet will also enable you to better manage your changing dietary requirements as you age. By being aware of your body, your awareness of what it needs and what food types don't work well will also increase. Hence, you'll become more effective in addressing changes in your metabolism; loss of taste sensation; the demands of medication and illness on your diet; and even alterations in your digestive system.

Difficulty chewing, having a dry mouth, and loss of appetite are pretty common in older adults. You'll be able to address these concerns more effectively through greater awareness of what you eat, ensuring your body still gets all the nutrients it needs.

Recommended Foods for a Mindful Diet

As you age, your digestive system may be unable to digest all kinds of food well. There may be certain foods that will benefit you more as they are easily digestible, helping your body gain all the nutrients it needs:

- **Plant-based foods** are rich in nutrients, offer lower calories than alternatives, and are easier to digest. These foods give your body the nutrients it needs without adding unnecessary calories that will only turn into fat as your body's energy requirement declines.
- **Whole foods** contain all the goodness nature intended without added preservatives and colorants. Including this kind of food can also prevent constipation due to its high fiber content, like salads, fresh fruit, and vegetables.
- **Nuts** are another great option as they're high in good fats that can help to combat cholesterol. For example, nuts are high in omega-3 fatty acids, contributing to brain health. Having a teaspoon of flaxseed oil daily can

also help you get enough good fats; such oils contain omegas: 3, 6, and 9.
- Always **drink enough water**. While a large part of our bodies consists of water, it also plays a vital role in ensuring bodily processes run smoothly. Water helps the body eliminate toxins, regulates body temperature, and improves circulation. With age, your body loses water which may cause you to feel thirsty less often. However, having approximately eight glasses of water daily is still essential.
- You can benefit from **limiting certain foods like coffee and red wine**. Remember that I said "limit" and not "exclude," as both these drinks benefit mature adults. Still, it would be best to enjoy them in moderation, which will become easier when you opt for mindful eating.
- Your **sugar intake is another concerning factor** to be aware of, as research indicates that sugar ages the body prematurely. This premature aging is linked to medical concerns like type 2 diabetes, certain cancers, and cardiovascular disease, all of which sugar contributes primarily to (Lam & Lam, n.d.).
- Many **overweight concerns happen due to mindless snacking** or eating so fast that your body doesn't realize it has had enough. When you choose to follow a mindful diet, you'll eat slower and with intention, being aware of all you eat. It will give your body plenty of time to realize it has had enough, and mindless snacking will disappear completely. This is also a way you can reduce your calorie intake without dieting.

- Trying to avoid or minimize **your red meat intake** will be beneficial. A far healthier option is lean meats that are hormone-free.
- Never neglect your **calcium intake** because this mineral is vital in mature adults to help preserve bone health. You won't have to take supplements when you include enough dairy products in your daily diet. Great alternatives, especially for those who struggle to digest cow's or goat's milk, are soy milk, and different types of nut milk like almond, cashew and coconut.

Foods That Boost Your Mood

You'll enjoy several outstanding benefits through proper diet management and mindful eating.

Several factors impact your energy level: not being active enough, not getting enough sleep, not being hydrated, and the food you eat. A persistent lack of energy and constantly feeling tired or foggy are sufficient reasons to be in a bad mood. However, these are all factors that are easy to manage.

Certain foods will help improve your mood through a mindful diet. When you include the following in your regular diet, it will bring a noticeable improvement to your mood (Davidson, 2020):

- Fatty fish is high in good fats like omega oils. These contribute to brain health by increasing the fluidity of your brain's cell membrane.

- Dark chocolate has become quite a topic of discussion since research reveals that dark and rich chocolate contains certain compounds that serve as mood boosters. It does this by supporting the release of several other compounds that will enhance your mood significantly.
- Fermented foods do wonders for your gut microbes, and the gut has increased in the importance allocated to it over the past couple of decades. Thanks to modern science, we know that gut health strongly impacts the brain and overall mood. Popular fermented food options are yogurt, kefir, sauerkraut, and kimchi.
- Bananas are a rich source of potassium that aids in muscle spasms, and it also has a lot of vitamin B6. The latter promotes the release of feel-good hormones such as dopamine.
- Oats are a whole food and high in fiber. The high fiber content of this much-loved breakfast option helps slow down the release of glucose into your blood and prevents sugar spikes followed by a low.
- Berries are high in antioxidants and linked to reduced depression symptoms and increased brain function.
- Nuts and seeds contain lots of tryptophan. Tryptophan is involved in the process of producing serotonin, which is another of the body's feel-good hormones.
- While you should always enjoy coffee in moderation—and it's best to have your last cup not late in the day, to keep the caffeine content from ruining a good night of sleep—it also aids in lifting your mood. The active ingredient in coffee increases the release of feel-good

hormones and prevents *adenosine*—a compound naturally present in the body—from attaching itself to brain receptors. By doing this, coffee helps you remain more alert and helps you maintain your focus.
- Beans and lentils are high in fiber and have lots of B vitamins. These vitamins improve neurological health and increase serotonin, dopamine, and other feel-good hormones.

These are some of the options you can choose from to improve your health and mood from the inside out every day! Remember, as important as it is to include all these foods, it's also important to refrain from overindulging. Always keep portion size in mind on your plate.

EXERCISING YOUR BRAIN

Maintaining a decent activity level will improve your overall wellness and mood. However, it's not only your body that needs exercise but your mind too. This will help you remain sharper, maintain your focus longer, and improve your memory when you include brain exercises in your regular routine. As a result, you'll also enjoy a far better mood. Some of the trusted brain exercise tools you can include in your life are right on your phone, and the following games are easy to download and play daily:

- **Sudoku:** This numbers game is a great exercise to improve short-term memory.
- **Luminosity:** It's easy to download this game onto your phone, and with a free account, you get three daily exercises to improve all brain functions through advanced mental activities.
- **Crosswords:** This is one of the oldest and most trusted brain exercises and helps to expand and maintain your verbal skills and aid memory.
- **Elevate:** This game offers a collection of brain training techniques suitable for a complete mental workout.
- **Peak:** Peak helps to improve mental agility, memory, focus, problem-solving skills, and much more.

Explore these and see what other brain games you can find that are both entertaining and offer your brain fun and challenging exercises.

LET'S GET PRACTICAL

Since mindfulness meditation is such a helpful aid in sustaining an overall sense of calm and greater joy and contentment, I want you to immerse yourself in the following exercise:

1. Settle in a comfortable position where you can sit undisturbed and relaxed for a while.
2. Decide on a set period of time you would like to meditate and set a timer.

3. Close your eyes and breathe deeply several times, taking note of how the air fills your lungs and causes your chest cavity to expand.
4. It can take a while to calm your mind, but just be kind to yourself. Whenever you wander off mentally, gently bring your thoughts back to the moment and your breath.
5. Become aware that in the present moment, there's nothing to fix, plan, stress about, or be scared of. It's a time when you can experience just being present in the moment.
6. Always return your thoughts to breathing and awareness of how clean air enters through your airways and unclean air escapes.
7. Once you're ready or your time has expired, gently open your eyes. Now you're prepared to take on your day with a much lighter and more relaxed approach.

You don't always have to sit and meditate to be mindful; you can also employ mindfulness in many daily tasks. The following exercise is one example of being mindful while doing a mundane task.

I call this exercise "wash and fold mindfully":

1. Before doing the laundry, take a few deep breaths and center your thoughts.
2. As you pick up every piece of laundry, notice the color and texture of the fabric.
3. Identify what sound you hear while doing your laundry.

4. When laundry is fresh out of the dryer, notice what you see, smell, and feel. Are the items still warm? Are they soft?
5. When you fold them, do so with care, noticing the finer details on the garments. If you can, try not to hurry through the task.
6. Once you are done, take a few deep breaths.

Answer the following questions:

- Was practicing this task hard or easy?
- How would you describe the quality of the experience?
- Did you feel any physical experiences while being mentally focused on only one task?

You can easily do the same when cooking food, cleaning the house, or washing the dishes.

BUSTING SIX AGING MYTHS

Through word of mouth and some media, several myths about aging have become so widely spread that many consider them to be truths.

Myth #1: It's Normal for Older People to Feel Depressed and Lonely

Truth

Studies reveal that the rate of depression is far higher in younger people than in more mature adults. Some older people may feel isolated due to specific circumstances that may result from a lack of mobility or medical condition, but it's not due to biological changes caused by getting older (National Institute on Aging, n.d.).

Myth #2: Older People Need Less Sleep

Truth

Older people may find it harder to fall asleep, and you'll need as many hours of sleep as any other adult.

Myth #3: Older People Struggle to Learn New Skills

Truth

As you age, the way you think and how your brain processes information may change, but you remain just as capable of learning new things as anyone else.

Myth #4: All Older People Get Dementia

Truth

Dementia is a mental concern and not a symptom of aging. All mature people tend to forget things sometimes, but these are—for most—merely occasional events, not dementia.

Myth #5: Older People Can Get Hurt When They Exercise

Truth

Anyone can get hurt when they start too fast or overdo it with too much exercise at once. Being active when you're older brings about many health benefits.

Myth #6: If One Family Member Has Alzheimer's Disease, All Are at Risk

Truth

Yes, certain genetic factors exist with this disease, but this is minimal and doesn't mean all family members are at risk, as several other factors can contribute to this diagnosis.

A FINAL WORD

- Happy and healthy aging occurs from the inside out. And the way you think, feel, eat, and perceive your life all contributes to your wellness.

- One of the benefits of aging is that after age 50, specific changes occur in your brain, allowing you to enjoy the benefits of an upwards happiness curve.
- Do you have a purpose? Having a purpose in midlife and onwards contributes to your mental and physical wellness.
- You can employ mindfulness to support your overall well-being. Consider mindfulness meditation, practicing mindful eating, and being conscious and aware of the present moment throughout your day.
- A mindful diet consists of foods that contribute to a good mood. It would also help to have sufficient sleep, exercise, and hydration to be happier too.
- Even when you mature, your brain still goes through developmental stages. Brain exercises can help you make the most of your neuroplasticity.
- Don't believe the myths about old age—chances are, they're only made-up stories.

STEPPING INTO YOUR AUTHENTIC SELF

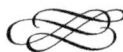

> *You can't help getting older, but you don't have to act old.*
>
> — GEORGE BURNS

For the longest time, you may have thought of yourself as an employee, boss, parent, child, sibling, spouse, or friend. However, these are all roles you fulfill and not your identity. Due to this confusion, it's easy to go through life without thinking about who you really are. However, when we grow older, and these roles aren't taking up as much time anymore, it can feel like we have lost ourselves. It can be a scary stage in life, but it's merely an illusion. If you think that way, it may not be because you're losing yourself but because you've never found your true identity.

LIVING AN AUTHENTIC LIFE

Life is short. Yet, it's never too late to get to know the person in the mirror. We can live an authentic life only when we're genuinely familiar with who we are.

There are several ways you can start living an authentic life or increase the level of authenticity in your life.

Understanding and Knowing What Your Core Values Are

We all have values, even though you might not have identified yours or think you value something but don't really. You will move one step closer to living an authentic life by defining your core values.

Your *core values* are those things that define you, how you live your life, what's acceptable to you, how you set your goals, and even what goals you set. Values are captured in one word, but the impact they have on your life is vast.

By knowing your values, you'll be able to make better choices and do so quickly and easily. Values offer greater clarity on where you want to invest your time and resources and where your obstacles are to achieving your goals. They'll even define what goals you set for yourself. Knowing your values makes you feel more confident, empowered, motivated, and at peace with who you are.

Have an Open Mind

When you live an authentic life, you do so based on your expectations of yourself rather than what you believe others want from you or think of you. What you think of yourself matters more than what others think of you. Through an open mind, you'll be able to notice wonderful opportunities. An open mind is also the key to including greater diversity in your life through the people you are friends with, as they'll be from all ages and walks of life, enriching your life.

Trust Your Gut

Living authentically gives you confidence in your gut feeling, as you know what's happening internally. Do regular introspections to determine your strengths and weaknesses and address any concerns while celebrating your strengths. Familiarizing yourself with who you are gives you trust in what you feel at your core.

There Will Be Resistance

In many parts of your life, you might have agreed to do things you didn't want to do. When you make a change and start to dance according to your own beat and not how others want you to dance, you may meet resistance. Therefore, protecting your values by setting boundaries is important to safely keep what's valuable to you.

LEARNING NEW THINGS

I can't recall ever being a fan of learning and getting acquainted with new skills. However, now I'm always keen on picking up a new skill as every skill I learn empowers me a little more, regardless of how old I am.

The most beneficial reason for investing time and effort in learning new skills is that it adds color to your life. And the most important reason to exert yourself to become familiar with a new trade, skill, or even language is that it brings several health benefits. Yes, can you believe it? Researchers recently determined that learning a new skill can improve your health as it keeps your brain busy and your mind sharp. Participants whose days were filled with many activities that kept them engaged and challenged them on several levels had far greater memory, were better at reasoning, had a much more advanced vocabulary, and their brain processes were much more developed compared to those whose days were mundane and empty (Providence Senior Health Team, 2020).

But how does learning new things truly benefit you? Suppose you're a literature fan of novels like *The Mill on the Floss*. In that case, you may be familiar with the name George Eliot, who was a woman called Mary Ann Evans. One of her famous quotes is: "It is never too late to be what you might have been" (Lisa, n.d., para. 4). I love this wisdom dating back to the 1800s.

Learning new skills in midlife and beyond can enhance your career. You may only need to add a certificate, course, or diploma to your name to take your career to the next level.

While it helps you to progress, learning new skills can also help you remain relevant. The pace at which technology developed over the past couple of centuries created an immense division between those keen to learn and adjust to the times and those who merely refused; the latter is irrelevant in the workplace today.

These skills can also help you discover new interests. All the advances I've mentioned are present in a range of fields, and not only are there many more passions to pursue, but old and familiar ones may also have developed entirely, making them far more interesting to you. However, it would help if you discovered them first; therefore, you need to be open to mastering new skills. This is a challenge, but as a result, you can be sure to enjoy greater mental agility and be much sharper. If your brain is a pencil, learning new skills surely is a sharpener, taking care to keep you in a mint state for as long as possible.

Making such progress and setting yourself apart from all others who refuse to exert themselves in this regard leaves you much more confident to approach even more significant challenges.

It's Never Too Late

Contrary to the popular belief that, at some point, you may be too old to learn, the reality is that as you age, your sense of responsibility, self-discipline, and comprehension of the world increases. Coupled with the fact that technology is making learning and accessing information so much easier today than ever before, you really should consider what's holding you back, for it's not due to your age.

What are some of the most common interests more mature adults pursue? Anything you like! And for inspiration, consider gardening, surfing, art, learning to play an instrument, getting familiar with a new language, or even taking up motorcycle riding like me!

AUTHENTICITY AND COMPASSION

One of the benefits of living an authentic life is that it becomes easier to be more compassionate. Compassion naturally grows with age, as we tend to be selfish and self-centered in our youth.

As we grow older and live more authentically, we grow more familiar with our failures, rejections, and heartache. The unpleasant experiences you have and the struggles you face leave you more in touch with the same battles others are facing, as well as feeling a far greater sense of compassion towards others. The same goes for empathy.

Empathy is also something you can increase by taking specific steps. These particular steps will help improve the quality of your authentic life too. Before going into that, I want to linger on what *empathy* is: It's the ability to immerse yourself into what another person is experiencing, that you feel their pain so vividly as if it's happening to you. Being empathetic doesn't mean that you crumble emotionally every time you observe someone else's pain, but that you have what is necessary to form solid foundations for relationships in your life—you have kindness and understanding, or "empathy."

We can also distinguish between *emotional empathy* and *cognitive empathy*. The first is very straightforward and refers to identifying with the emotions others experience and feeling compassion towards them. The second relates to understanding why someone feels a certain way and behaves in a specific manner. It doesn't mean you agree with the way they behave, but you have compassion for what they're experiencing and understand why they may act out.

How does this even happen that you feel someone else's pain without experiencing what they experience? Professional experts believe this is possible due to our ability to simulate what others are going through. This simulation—called the *simulation theory*—enables us to vividly imagine our emotions responding similarly. This effect is coupled with "mirror neurons" in the human brain, allowing us to activate and experience similar emotions to what we see.

Increase Your Ability to Experience Empathy

For some, empathy comes quite naturally, and you can also enhance the degree to which you experience it:

- **Show interest in others:** Most people are keen to talk about themselves, and you won't have to nudge them to open up to you if they can see you're authentic in your empathy and want to help them. Be curious about what people are doing and why they behave in a specific manner without being nosey. Showing interest in other people's stories will widen your perspective of the world.

- **Zoom in on similarities:** It can be easy to get bogged down by how people differ from you. They may have different cultures and religions or be from different races, but ultimately we are all human, which ties us all together. Explore how others are similar to you and how they feel the same pain, frustration, anger, and disappointment as you, rather than how they may look or talk differently from you.
- **Imagine being in someone else's shoes:** You may never know exactly how someone else is feeling, but you can get quite close by visualizing yourself in their situation and how you would feel if it was you. This keeps volunteers passionate about making a time investment in the lives of others.
- **Listen and share:** You'll find that often, the best thing you can do is just listen to what others have to say. It may be that they don't feel heard or want to get something off their chest. And you can also share your experiences as these events make you more relatable, increase their trust in you, and determine how much they are willing to share with you.
- **Go beyond one-on-one interaction:** You can also increase your empathy through group exposure. Social platforms can be a great way to share encouragement and advice and show that you care and are willing to offer support.
- **Be creative:** People are around you every day who are facing challenges, experiencing hardship, and feeling

sorrow, but you'll never know without communicating through a smile, making eye contact, or simply asking how they're doing. Why not try this next time when you fill up your car, buy groceries, or go for a walk?

The Outcome of Compassion and Empathy Is Genuine Connections

Genuine connections refer to those moments when the masks come off, and we're honest with each other, regardless of how ugly the truth may be. It takes place when you have such a strong bond that you know the other person accepts you for who you are, warts and all, and you don't have to hide behind a façade. These are highly enriching connections to have. They become vital in midlife and beyond because they fill your days, keep you busy, and give you purpose.

However, genuine connections require patience as they take time to form. Nonetheless, there are specific steps you can take to create these bonds:

- **Just show up:** It's often the case that you don't have to say or do much—you just need to be there. Be with someone, sit with them without saying or doing anything. People are social beings, and our emotional burden becomes lighter when shared with another.
- **Listen attentively:** It's not always the case that the other person wants to share what they have on their mind, or it may take a little time for them to open up. When they do, you need to listen attentively. Please

don't interrupt or tell them what they should've or shouldn't have done. Just listen without judgment, taking in all they communicate verbally and through non-verbal clues like facial expressions and body language.

- **Ask questions to gain a better understanding:** Without prying into their lives, you can show interest and curiosity in their situation by asking questions that will give you greater clarity.
- **Show empathy:** The best way to identify what action you need to take is to show that you care by putting yourself in their situation and then deciding what you would want the other person to do. This will help you to take the correct action.
- **No motives:** You should have no ulterior reasons when listening during these moments. It's not about judging and getting fresh gossip. Conversations between people with genuine connections are private and should always take place in a safe space.

CREATING MORE GENUINE CONNECTIONS

Having genuine connections can benefit you in multiple ways and helps you gain several such relationships. And, when you are keen to create more of these bonds, it's important to never rely on these relationships when it comes to your well-being or your happiness. True happiness comes from within and isn't anchored in any relationship. These also differ from relationships that are always smooth sailing and feel good. The deeper the connections are, the more likely there will be challenges, and by overcoming these challenges, you'll grow closer. These challenges result from the fact that both parties are deeply invested in this bond compared to superficial connections with minimal investment.

To prevent these challenges from becoming destructive, you should set specific boundaries. While your happiness should never be rooted in these relationships, you should also not allow the nature of the connection to negatively impact your happiness. Boundaries don't mean that you block people out of your life, only that you let them into your life in an acceptable manner for both.

Another sign of a genuine connection is that it doesn't always mean you have to talk. Sometimes, you can just be in the moment, sharing the present without saying anything. It's the kind of relationship that demands both parties give and take without co-dependency. Since you'll be putting yourself in a vulnerable position, which may be risky, you may need to be vulnerable to be daring and courageous. Still, it would help if you always remain responsible for this choice and any other actions you take or things you say. So, if you were vulnerable and then scorned, you still have to acknowledge that you took a risk and were brave, but it didn't work out as you envisioned.

Ultimately, these are the kind of relationships you should value the bond and the person and not what you can gain from it. It's a bond where you'll give and receive love, and you should always approach it with kindness and respect.

In our youth, it was easy to have friendships rooted in mere convenience. In our older years, it's a different story; we seek connections rather than convenience, when we no longer want to waste time on superficial bonds or feel we need to keep up a façade. Thus, forming and strengthening genuine connections becomes much more critical as we age.

VOLUNTEERING AND MENTORING

I've touched on the benefits of volunteering and how it can add purpose to your life. It's also a fantastic way to form strong bonds and increase your sense of authenticity. Consider volunteering anytime in your life and even more so after retirement. You could find yourself in a position where you've been looking forward to those lazy days when you don't have to rush off to work, sit in the traffic, or have little time to do everything you want to do. But, perhaps soon after retirement, you became bored and can't remember why you craved so much free time anymore.

This is when you should get your name on a list seeking relief offered by volunteers, as volunteering provides the following benefits:

- It offers a sense of community, helping you feel part of something larger than your own life.
- Meeting up with others in this regard becomes a social event, keeping you mentally, emotionally, and physically fit.
- It adds a sense of purpose to your life, leaving you feeling satisfied and confident that you make a difference in the lives of others and the world.

- This is not to make money—there might even be a minor financial investment from you—but the return on your investment is far too valuable to ever be measured in monetary gain.

Tips on Finding the Right Volunteer Opportunity for You

Becoming a volunteer is often a long-term commitment. The following tips will help you make a choice that's sustainable for you:

- Don't overcommit your time. You may be amped up initially, but manage your time so it's not consumed by volunteering.
- It shouldn't be a hassle, as it may rob you of the pleasures you gain from the process.
- Be discerning in your choice. Not all opportunities are equally rewarding. Choose well where you want to get involved.
- Know yourself and what you like and also what you don't like. This will help you find something that complements your identity.
- If you're checking a volunteer opportunity out, make it clear from the start that you're looking for the best option.

When you've found the right option, it can be a mutually beneficial arrangement that allows you to pass on your knowledge and skills to the next generations. This is especially true if you prefer to work with younger people who are interested in finding a mentor to guide them along in life. If you choose to contribute to the lives of others your age, you can get involved in efforts where you'll collaborate with your peers. Or, if you prefer to work with those older than yourself, it's an excellent way to gain insight and knowledge from the older generation's journeys.

POSITIVE EMOTIONS LEAD TO POSITIVE HEALTH

When you go through stages of high stress, sadness, rejection, or any other negative emotion, it has an impact on your physical health. This impact can be so severe that chronic stress can shorten your lifespan. At the core of this rippling effect is how negative emotions influence hormonal balance. At the same time, chronically elevated stress levels cause high blood pressure, heart disease, and even digestive concerns (Lawson, n.d.). While life is far more pleasant when we're happy and content, the need to be positive is further enhanced by the positive impact of feeling good on your physical being.

When you encourage positive emotions in your life, you will be able to expand your perspective on the world. It awakens the need to be more creative as getting lost in the wonder surrounding you is easier. Lasting positive emotions also leads to greater emotional resiliency which helps you overcome emotionally turbulent times more quickly.

Being more positive is more challenging than it sounds, as it entails overcoming negative biases. Negative bias refers to those times when you choose to remain vigilant, always expecting the other shoe to drop. Sure, many bad things happen in the world and even in our lives, but expecting the next bad thing to occur, robs you of happiness and isn't a healthy approach to life either. The negativity of such a bias severely impacts your life, and for every instance you give it the lead, you need three cases of positivity to balance out the effect (Lawson, n.d.).

Another approach to overcome negative bias is to forgive. Through forgiveness, you can accept that something terrible has happened and, through this acceptance, you can move forward. Forgiveness doesn't mean what was done to you was right; instead, you will no longer tie yourself down by not letting go. Researchers also indicate that forgiveness can reduce feeling hurt by as much as 70%; minimize anger by 13%; and drop the number of complaints you have against the other person or situation by 27% (Lawson, n.d.).

By having greater positivity in your life, you become more like an emotional rubber band, able to restore your shape even when you've been under pressure of obstacles challenging you emotionally.

LET'S GET PRACTICAL

It's time for some love and kindness towards yourself and others. Amplifying these positive emotions is at the core of loving-kindness meditation. You can follow the same steps in the mindfulness meditation explained in the previous chapter. However, now your focus will be on practicing self-compassion:

1. First, reach out to the deepest parts of your being and connect with yourself. Explore how you feel, what you think, and what you desire for yourself now. What's bothering you or hurting you? You can repeat positive and comforting statements like: "May I be healthy," May I be happy," and "May I be content."
2. From here onwards, expand your focus to a friend or a family member you care deeply about. Visualize the person being happy, healthy, content, and successful. See how their dreams become a reality. Enjoy the moment while repeating phrases like: "May you be healthy," "May you be happy," and "May you be content."
3. The world is full of people, and they aren't all friends or loved ones. Some are mere strangers. Yet, you can connect with them too. It could be someone you often see in the street but have never met. Now visualize this person and see them in a state of happiness and health. Use similar phrases as before.
4. Lastly, the world also has its share of difficult people. You might not know why they're complicated, but you want to reach out to them in kindness. Visualize your desire for them to be happy, content, and healthy while using the same phrases.

Afterward, reflect on your experience and answer the following questions:

- How did it feel to be compassionate towards yourself?
- When will you set aside time in your day to practice self-compassion?

- How did you feel when you visualized compassion towards others?
- How can you become more compassionate towards others and yourself?

Next, compile a list of all your relationships, from family and friends to coworkers and even beyond:

- Identify the relationships you consider authentic, and express gratitude for having these people in your life.
- Identify what relationships you would like to grow stronger and how you can make an effort to strengthen these bonds.
- Schedule time to meet more people in person next week rather than online.

A FINAL WORD

- The older we get, the more crucial it is to get truly familiar with ourselves and to know our identity. This is how we create and build an authentic life, and it's a way of living with multiple benefits.
- While it's often assumed older people can't learn new skills, this notion is merely a myth. Learning new skills is possible and highly beneficial as we age.
- Investing in yourself to learn new skills is a form of self-compassion, and you can also learn to have more compassion and empathy toward others. Both of these will help you form authentic bonds that add value to

your life and offer an opportunity to add value to the lives of others.
- These bonds allow you to enjoy genuine connections and find purpose in helping others. Volunteering is a fantastic way to increase the number of these connections in your life.
- Volunteering adds meaning and purpose to your life and leaves you feeling positive. Positive emotions are a vital supplement to sustain good physical health.

HELPING SOMEONE ELSE TO TAKE THEIR FIRST STEP

"Helping others, without expecting anything in return is what true self-worth is all about."

— GAVIN BIRD

Perhaps you remember that in the introduction, I mentioned the value I found in helping others – how it added meaning to my life (and still does).

Much as it was important for me to do things for myself to add that value to my life, helping other people is still an important factor. In fact, studies show that volunteering and giving to just causes improves both emotional and physical health.

It activates positive emotions and reduces negativity, supporting your well-being… and amazingly enough, it also strengthens your immune system and enhances your body's ability to function.

So while doing things that would enable me to inhabit and express my authentic self has been an important part of my journey, doing things for other people is still key.

I'd like to invite you to do that now… And the best part is, you don't even need to leave your sofa.

Writing this book was my way of helping other women to weave the gold into their golden years… and you can join me in my mission by writing a short review.

By leaving a review of this book on Amazon, you'll show new readers where they can find the guidance they're looking for to make sure they age well and live their best life, no matter the number of candles on the cake.

Simply by letting other women know how this book has helped you and what they'll find within its pages, you'll provide a signpost that shows them where they can find the help they're looking for.

Thank you so much for your support. When you take the right approach, every single part of your day can add value to your life… and by joining me on my mission, you'll not only add value to yours; you'll help other people too.

STEP UP AND LOVE YOURSELF

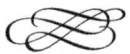

> *Years may wrinkle the skin, but to give up interests, wrinkle the soul. You are as young as your faith, as old as your doubts; as young as your self-confidence, as old as your fears, as young as your hopes, and as old as your despairs.*
>
> — DOUGLAS MACARTHUR

As we go through life, the number of times we experience heartache, disappointment, loss, rejection, hurt, financial despair, or trauma increases. Every time something like this happens, it impacts our confidence and diminishes our hopes for the future. Even worse is when we overcome the setback and find joy, hope, peace, or stability again when such events occur; we experience these joyful moments with a sense of fear caused by the question of when the second shoe will drop. How soon will we lose it all again?

This way of thinking is the breeding ground of self-doubt, robbing you of the joy you should be experiencing during your golden years. It's easy to allow yourself to shift into a *scarcity mindset*, a post-traumatic stress response to the live events you've endured. Yet, suppose you don't actively work to overcome this mindset. In that case, you are diminishing the quality of life you could be experiencing.

BECOMING VISIBLE AGAIN

You'll find negative thought patterns at the center of the whirlwind of self-doubt causing chaos in your life. Realizing how impactful your thoughts are and how they contribute to your overall happiness is the first step to freedom and joy. When you have control over your thoughts, you can determine what kinds of thoughts you want to host and take the steps needed to break free from any negative thoughts:

- **Acknowledge your negative thoughts**. Negative thoughts are something everyone is struggling with, and you can't deny them. The first step to addressing these thoughts is to acknowledge their existence and that you have them.
- **Compare your current situation to previous situations**. When have you experienced the same doubts as now? How did that situation turn out? The outcome of the last time you were in a similar situation can bring you comfort and understanding in the present moment.

- **Stop comparing your life with those of others**. The lives of others may appear to be better than yours, but you only know half of their story. You have no idea what their situation is.
- **Add gratitude to your life**. Doubt disappears in the light of gratitude.
- **Stop yourself from worrying about what others think**. People don't think as much about you as you may think, and what they believe about you should never out weigh more than what you know about yourself.
- **Surround yourself with people who uplift and inspire you**. You can also gain positivity by listening to uplifting podcasts and reading books that help you have a better life.
- **You Shouldn't take everything personally**. People say things and behave in a manner that might be offensive or hurtful. What caused them to behave this way probably has nothing to do with you and is perhaps linked to what they're going through.

Due to the increased number of setbacks you might have experienced in your life, it can be harder to control negative thinking and overcome self-doubt. Therefore, as you age, you can also incorporate these steps to help you to keep self-doubt at bay:

- **Find support from other women sharing your sentiments in women's circles**. By joining these types of groups, you can surround yourself with like-minded

people willing to uplift you and become your support network.
- **Don't allow self-doubt to limit your life**. Do you want to start surfing, learn to play an instrument, or master a new language? Does self-doubt present itself as fear about what others would think, or do you feel you'll make a fool of yourself? Face your fears and do it anyway!
- **Trust that everything is in your favor** and nobody wants to see you fail.
- **Celebrate your small victories in life**. It may appear insignificant to others when you've managed to hold your breath underwater for more than two minutes, but it may be a breakthrough for you. So celebrate all your victories because each one will help you reach your next goal.
- **Doubting yourself, your abilities, or your choices is part of any stage of life**. During your teenage years, you may have struggled with pimples. While it was awful to look at yourself in the mirror and only see all those blemishes on your skin, you knew the problem would eventually improve or naturally disappear when you became older. Self-doubt is different; you need to address it to rid yourself of its limitations in your life. Start right away by making this day a confident one with some positive affirmations.

BECOME VISIBLE

Do you feel invisible? Maybe you've been so busy helping everyone else that you've lost your identity? Too many women settle for being the cement in life. What do I mean by "cement"? Let me explain. Visualize a magnificent mosaic wall. Passersby admire the beauty of the tile work, the distinctive patterns, and how it all comes together to create an impressive piece of art. Does anyone ever comment on the cement holding these tiles into place on the wall? No, of course not. People don't even notice the cement or acknowledge the contribution it makes.

You might have been so busy helping others to shine for the longest time that you forgot you have a right to shine too. Thus, you've become invisible to the world. You might have only realized that you were in this state once the kids left home or when you entered menopause. Perhaps a clerk in a store walked right past you to help a much younger lady who had just entered, or when you were overlooked for a promotion year after year after being told you weren't experienced enough. Then the story turns out that you're not young enough. Why doesn't anyone see you? Is it because you're invisible?

One way you can turn the light onto yourself and enjoy the attention you deserve is to P.R.E.P.A.R.E. Yes, you can prepare yourself to overcome your invisibility:

- **Posture:** Enter any room or conversation like a queen. Do you need encouragement to become a queen-ager? Place your hands on your hips with your feet shoulder-

width apart, chest out, chin up, and think of an invisible cape billowing out behind you!
- **Renovate:** When was the last time you renovated your appearance? There's no need for plastic surgery—try changing your hair, makeup, or wardrobe and experience the difference.
- **Educate:** Learn a new skill or stay on track with modern advancements.
- **Passion:** What inspires you and wakes you up inside? What's one thing you can do for hours and still not feel exhausted? Do more of those things.
- **Attitude:** Are you a chronic downer? It's often the case that people treat us the way we teach them to treat us. Change your mindset and re-educate those who surround you.
- **Relationships:** Embrace those in your community. Listen to the many stories people share during your day. Make new friends and strengthen your bonds.
- **Energize:** It's time to take action by being active. The more active you are, the more your energy level will increase.

You deserve to be a queen-ager, so wear your invisible cape with confidence, and you will become all that you set out to be!

CHANGE YOUR THOUGHTS AND INCREASE YOUR RESILIENCE

Why is it that negative thinking is so common among older adults? After all, you may feel that you've seen it all at your age and should know better. But still, you can't escape the dark cloud hanging over your head, tainting your perspective on everything with a shade of darkness. Maybe it's because of the many failures you endured, but there's more to it. Let's dig into some of the most predominant causes of negative thinking patterns.

When you see life as black or white, wrong or right, it's tough to avoid negativity, as you allow no room for anything in-between. I'm referring not only to moral principles and values but also to those instances where you just gave up on something or someone because you didn't get it perfect the first time. Give yourself a break, Woman! Life has many shades and tones for you to enjoy:

- **Overgeneralization robs you of all joy**. Something might have happened once, and now you believe it will happen in the same manner all the time, or one person behaved in a particular way. You may think all similar people will act the same.
- **Your mental filter might only allow you to see all that is wrong or not right**. Only you can change your mental settings to make room for positivity.
- **When you do notice the positive, you devalue it**. Celebrate all things positive, and they will multiply.
- **How often do you jump to conclusions?** How often are your decisions wrong? Think about how much time you've wasted by doing this.
- **You are prone to exaggeration**. The opposite can also be the case. Always ask yourself what you believe has

supporting evidence or facts backing up your beliefs. If not, it's time to change your perceptions.

- **Believing everything you are feeling can be self-destructive.** You feel scared about taking a big step, and now you've chosen to believe that you'll make a mistake. This cognitive distortion keeps you stagnant—more on that soon.
- **You think there are certain things you should do as they are expected of you.** Have you ever asked yourself, is this the right thing to do? And does it make sense? If not, why do it?
- **You label yourself based on your actions.** You might have made a mistake by having too much to drink at a get-together. It may be because you're a light drinker, not because of what others may think of you, causing you to label yourself an "embarrassing drinker."
- **You place all the blame on yourself.** You don't have control over everything; therefore, you're not responsible for everything. Stop blaming yourself or thinking you're always coming up short.

When negative thinking becomes part of a much bigger and more intrinsic network, you're looking at cognitive distortion and its negative impact on your life. The term *cognitive distortion* refers to when the negative thoughts in your mind are distorting reality, leaving you in a desperate state of anxiety and depression, while the ideas that placed you in this state are far removed from reality.

Cognitive Distortion

Being an overthinker is one of the most prominent causes leading to cognitive distortion. Are you a person who obsesses over every little detail or what might go wrong? When you're at the center of this overthinking and persistent in obsessing over your flaws—thus gradually expanding them in your mind—then this kind of rumination will also contribute to cognitive distortion. The final cause of this concern directs the negativity that's present away from yourself and towards others. In short, you perceive the world and everyone in it with disdain, mistrust, and even anger. It truly sucks to spend your golden years immersed in such dark negativity when this should be the best time ever. Please don't fret too much, as you can break this negative thought chain.

How do I ever do that? You may be asking yourself.

Sometimes, the more you push negative thinking out of your mind, the more those ideas will pop right back in with even greater force. So, give these thoughts some airtime, but limit these thoughts to a very brief time in your day. Then, ask them to leave! And whenever these negative thoughts surface again and again, try replacing them with positive thoughts again and again. If negative thoughts aren't going away, you can also place them on hold to cover during a specific time of day. Once you've moved negative thoughts to wait in line at your negative thinking window, replace them with positive ones. The more you do this exercise, the more you'll find these negative thoughts moving outside your mind.

Do you love yourself? Self-love is one of the most undervalued solutions to ending negative thoughts. Essentially, negative thoughts are nothing but negative self-talk. This isn't how you would talk to a loved one, so why do you speak to yourself this way when loving yourself? Self-love can nip negative thinking in the bud.

Keep a journal; this is a great place to write about all the positive things that happen in your daily life! It can also be a place to record all the beauty you notice in your surroundings.

Be careful of what you give an entry pass into your thoughts. Are you allowing social media or even the news to drop all the bad happening in the world into your mind? Would you allow the garbage truck to dump the garbage of the entire neighborhood on your front porch? Obviously not, so stop allowing the media to drop the dirt of the world where you must mentally process several nasties that far exceed any person's capacity. Try cutting down on the time you spend absorbing the news by exercising or meditating.

WHAT IS YOUR PERSPECTIVE ON AGING?

Do you suffer from *ageism*—a negative perspective on growing older? In essence, ageism is no different than racism and sexism. It places a negative and unfair attitude on a specific group, causing unfair treatment based on a particular factor. If you're suffering from ageism, it will impact your life negatively too. Your focus will be on the negative aspects of growing older while failing to see all the pros of reaching this stage in life. It will also make you dread growing older, a part of life you simply can't escape from.

You can overcome this bias by exploring the *positive aging movement*. This refers to adopting a positive perspective on aging despite certain factors like fading health, slower movement, and deteriorating memory. It demands that you give more attention to all that can be good and manifest these things in your life.

Pursue positive aging by keeping fit—physically and mentally—changing your lifestyle to complement your age, maintaining strong bonds, and creating positive experiences.

Remaining positive while experiencing all these changes demands greater resilience in life. And this is something you can master now.

You can rewrite your story, regardless of your age. Recapture your past by changing your perspective; from this foundation, it will be easier to change the direction of your future. When you ponder your story, remember all the times you faced adversity and how you overcame it successfully. Resilience can also increase when you offer support to others, thus offering a lending hand or simply an ear willing to listen when needed. You'll notice that you can handle far more if you give yourself time to take breaks in between. Breaks don't have to be long; ensure they're regular to help you continue easily. Lastly, stepping outside your comfort zone increases your familiarity with what's unknown and allows you to practice resilience in a controlled manner.

SELF-PRAISE

Nobody likes someone who's constantly blowing their own horn, but that isn't the same as self-praise. If you have a different idea of what self-praise means, it can rob you of the benefits this action offers.

Self-praise is an effective way to increase your self-esteem and confidence in order to tackle new challenges with vigor and anticipation. If done correctly, self-praise can establish your reputation as someone who's capable, trustworthy, and respected. It can change the entire way others perceive you and treat you. If you hide your accomplishments and never share your successes, you're not the only person at a loss here. You're also withholding others from getting to know the real you and how you can add value to their lives.

Positive Affirmations to Lift Your Mood

We've already touched on the power of positive affirmations and how they can improve your life. When it comes to overcoming negativity, positive affirmations also have a valuable role to play as a reminder that life is good, and the more you focus and visualize the good, the more it will multiply and manifest in your life.

Some of my favorite positive affirmations that I say daily are:

- "I am so proud of my long and healthy life."
- "I am happy and content in my home environment."

- "I enjoy the benefits of experience and wisdom in my life."
- "I know I can do anything I set my mind to."

What are some positive affirmations you would like to say and visualize daily?

POSITIVE ATTITUDES

You can also include kindness to help you become more positive. To truly benefit from including kindness in your life, understand kindness as more than an adverb describing an action; see it as a verb. Therefore, you can refer to kindness as art with specific helpful attributes.

Kindness supports mental health and increases the secretion of feel-good hormones like serotonin and dopamine (Siegle, 2020). While these endorphins do wonders for your mood, they're also great painkillers, and you can find pain relief by showing compassion to others.

It's also great for your physical health as it decreases the release of *cortisol*, the stress hormone that causes havoc on your overall wellness. If cortisol remains persistently present at high levels, it can cause high blood pressure, heart disease, strokes, and even diabetes (Siegle, 2020).

Another vital characteristic of kindness is that it exceeds how you treat others and demands that you're also kind to yourself. It entails giving yourself the grace to relax, stop beating yourself up over mistakes you've made—because you're only human—and know when to release some steam to release the tension, heartache, or any other negative emotions building up internally.

Kindness demands you get off your laurels and start acting by practicing compassion toward others. Help where you can, contribute to solutions, take action that aids the environment, volunteer, take up a hobby, or do whatever is necessary to be a better version of yourself towards others and yourself.

It will ease the pain and discomfort of growing older. The more you lose your physical youth and mental clarity, the more you need to silence the inner critic reminding you of your failures or how you can no longer do what you wanted to do. Kindness is the foundation of self-compassion, the antidote to the self-inflicted pain of our choices and what we put ourselves through mentally, emotionally, and physically (Intermountain Health Care, 2019).

A counterpart to kindness in your quest for greater positivity in your life is gratitude. I've already said a lot about gratitude, and I want to remind you that gratitude has a domino effect on your life. Once you actively start practicing gratitude—whether by keeping a gratitude journal, posting notes of thanks into a gratitude jar, or choosing gratitude meditation—it impacts your life in several ways.

You will experience improved health and wellness mentally, physically, and emotionally, and you'll also notice your relationships becoming healthier and stronger. Happiness increases, and so does your ability to apply self-control. Gratitude is one of the primary building blocks to enjoying a higher quality of life (Siegle, 2020).

WHY SELF-CARE IS VITAL AS YOU AGE

You're no longer a spring chicken. You're a queen-ager enjoying the golden years of your life. What are you waiting for to start taking care of yourself? And, if you won't take care of yourself in the most intimate way, who will? While you're probably in the stage of your life where you have more time than ever to invest in self-care, it's also more crucial than before to do so now. It's vital to prioritize your health, fitness, mental state, and emotional well-being; cherish your dreams; and realize your goals.

Suppose you've considered self-care a mere spoil for selfish people. In that case, it might be harder to make the mental shift into making self-care a priority, and it may be even harder to determine where you need to start:

- **Self-care is more than regular trips to the salon** to take care of your nails or hair—those are treats you deserve too. However, at the foundation of self-care, you'll find that it entails letting go of the guilt of your past. This burden is too heavy to carry any further into your future. Now's the time to accept that there are certain things you can't change and you aren't doing anyone any favors by carrying the emotional burden. Accept what has happened and kiss guilt goodbye.

- **Being more active is another way to take care of yourself.** There may have been times when you wanted to exercise but didn't allow yourself to fit this into your schedule. Your needs deserve priority, and it's time to get active now.
- **Embrace what you feel.** Do you find something funny? Then laugh until your entire body is shaking. Spend time with people who make you laugh and with who you like to be silly. Life is too short to be serious all the time.
- **Eat well and indulge in healthy foods.** Hydrate enough and be kind to your body by giving it what it needs. Remember that getting enough quality sleep, regardless of your age, is one of the most beneficial favors you can do yourself.
- **Look in the mirror and express love towards the image you see**, for this is you—amazing, incredible you!

It's easier to make self-care part of your life when you create a routine around the practices you want to include.

By drafting a specific routine, you show the intent of kindness towards yourself, and by following your routine diligently, you're committing to your well-being. What will your plan include? The titles of the books you want to read? A creative project you want to get your hands on? Salsa classes or any other forms of fun activities? Whatever you want to do, get going and start taking care of yourself!

LET'S GET PRACTICAL

Gratitude is such a significant component of being more positive about life. Are you ready to take on this routine?

For the next week, commit to writing 10 things you're grateful for daily. Try refraining from repeating stuff you've already listed. By the end of the week, you'll be aware of 70+ reasons to smile and be happy. Note how doing this changes your life.

A FINAL WORD

- Love yourself. Please do it now and do it deeply. You can crush self-doubt and become the queen-ager you're always meant to be. While it may be harder to make this shift when you're older, I've shared several tips to make this task easy to accomplish.
- Several factors contribute to negative thinking and negatively will impact your overall wellness. By changing your way of thinking, you can overcome this hurdle that keeps you from living the life you desire and helps you gain greater resilience.
- *Ageism* is a negative bias towards growing older that will rob you of your joy. Do what's necessary to combat this as soon as you recognize that it's in your life.
- Self-praise, when done appropriately, is doing yourself a favor and helping others know and appreciate you more.
- Kindness is an act that goes beyond being nice to others —you also need to be kind to yourself. Investing time

and effort into self-care is one of the most effective ways to show compassion to yourself while enjoying all the benefits it brings.

STEPPING INTO PHYSICAL AND SOCIAL ACTIVITIES

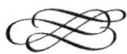

> *Age is not lost youth but a new stage of opportunity and growth.*
>
> — BETTY FRIEDAN

I want to emphasize the importance of staying fit as you grow older. However, when I use the word "fit," I mean both physically and socially. Let's explore physical fitness first.

THE BENEFITS OF EXERCISE

Even if you're only capable of small movements, it's vital that you still make the most of it. While staying fit is beneficial throughout your entire life, it's a matter of even greater urgency when you're older. Regular exercise helps improve balance which can prevent nasty falls and injuries. It's also an effective way to combat declining energy levels and prevent different types of diseases. Furthermore, you can also help your brain remain sharp longer since there's a strong link between physical and mental fitness. Several studies show a reduced risk of dementia and increased cognitive functioning in older adults who remain physically active (The Greenfields Continuing Care Community, n.d.).

Exercise can also be used to remain socially active, as you can join a club where like-minded people gather. Examples of such clubs are hiking, pickleball, and gardening clubs, to name a few. However, this can also take on a less formal format as you may even belong to a group of friends who meet regularly for a brisk walk.

WHAT IS MINDFUL MOVEMENT?

While "mindful movement" might be unfamiliar to you, you'll find the names of more familiar activities under this umbrella term. I'm referring specifically to yoga and tai chi. *Mindful movement* is an exercise aimed at getting your body moving, increasing circulation, and using your breathing to calm your mind and help you enter a state of complete relaxation. While practicing these exercises, you reduce negative emotions, release stress, and encourage healing.

More on Tai Chi

Tai Chi isn't the kind of exercise where you'll be doing any jumps, squats, or even lifting weights, but don't underestimate it as a potent exercise. Research shows that by regularly practicing this type of mindful movement, you can improve your balance, your agility and minimize joint pain. This is a practical activity for older adults and is even a safe option for those with Parkinson's disease. As you grow older, the risk of falling becomes more significant, and it can eventually become a concern of such severity that you may start to move around less often, as the fear that you may fall is so overpowering. Here too, Tai Chi is a fantastic solution—it reduces the chances of falling and the anxiety of it happening (Stelter, 2022).

Tai Chi is usually practiced in a group setting—an opportunity to remain socially active too—and if you can't find any clubs near you, you'll be able to get training online, which gives you the option to try it in the comfort of your home.

Fall Prevention Exercises

The following exercises can also help you improve your balance and prevent falls and the long recovery that often occurs after these types of injuries:

- chair sit-to-stand exercises
- side leg raises while holding on to the top of a chair
- back leg raises while holding onto the back of a chair
- heel-to-toe while standing

- heel-to-toe walks
- side twists while standing
- side twists on one leg
- marching in one place

Other Exercise Options

There are quite a few exercise options specifically aimed at older women. See if you can find any places in your community offering any of the following, and then watch how your overall health improves:

- Water aerobics allows for a good workout without the risk of injury.
- Yoga makes for a great mindful exercise that can be easily accessible from your home or in a gym.
- Resistance band workouts enable you to better manage your exercise level.
- Pilates is great for developing pelvic strength and is a trusted way to address concerns like incontinence.
- Walking is an excellent option. Try making it an event by enjoying your surroundings or spending time in nature.
- Body weight workouts can help you increase overall muscle mass.
- Dumbbell strength training is also an excellent way to increase strength, but please start slowly and with the guidance of a qualified fitness instructor to prevent injury.

However, suppose you've been fit your entire life or have worked on your strength and resilience for a while already; then you should be able to partake in more challenging exercises. I'm referring to the following:

- rock climbing
- long-distance running
- leg presses
- bench presses
- crunches
- rowing
- squats with dumbbells
- deadlifting
- high-intensity interval training (HIIT)

Exercising Tips

It doesn't matter what type of exercise you choose. What's important is that you exercise in a safe environment, never exert yourself to the extent of risking injury, and make this part of your regular schedule.

To enjoy the ultimate benefits of walking, try reaching a goal of 150 minutes per week. This can easily be broken down into 30-minute walks, 5 days a week. You can also break this down into 2 longer sessions or try hiking for 75 minutes at a time.

For those who need to work on their balance, an easy solution is to stand as much as you can on one leg, holding your balance for as long as possible. Remember to rotate your legs to give both legs a good workout.

Getting rid of excess weight, losing bone density and muscle mass, and poor posture are all common concerns for older adults. You can also improve these concerns by doing two to three hours of weight training weekly (National Institute on Aging, n.d.).

Before deciding on what kind of exercise would be best suited for you, consider the following points:

- Will it be fun? For any activity to be sustainable, you should enjoy what you're doing. This will help you be active on days when motivation is not enough to get you there.
- It's important you choose an option that's an easy fit for your lifestyle. You should be able to do this conveniently, and it won't clash with your other responsibilities.
- Keep a journal of your exercise progress, especially during those much harder early days. This will give you a record of how much you've progressed since you started.
- If you have any medical concerns—or any concerns at all regarding your planned exercise routine—see your healthcare professional first. Prevention remains the best option, and getting the green light from a medical expert before making any drastic changes that may impact your health is always a great thing to do.
- Suppose you're struggling with severe stiffness, pain, or discomfort. In that case, scheduling an appointment with a physician, chiropractor, or massage therapist will

be beneficial. These healthcare professionals will be able to bring the relief you seek, and they can offer advice on how you should proceed.
- The most important tip to remember is to have fun and remember to drink plenty of water before, during, and after each exercise routine. Exercise doesn't have to be a burden. You'll see that the more you enjoy what you're doing, the easier it will be to keep up this healthy habit.

STAYING SOCIALLY FIT

Physical activity is just one form of exercise you need. It would help if you're also a fit communicator in order to strengthen your social bonds. Familiarizing yourself with mindful communication will provide a greater interest for your presence in social circles. It will also enable you to reap all the benefits I've mentioned earlier that are linked to deep and meaningful relationships.

Mindful communication refers to far more than being an eloquent speaker. It also means you're comfortable with being an active listener. While active listeners soak up all the words the other person is saying, they actively observe the speaker's facial expressions, body language, posture, and nonverbal clues. Spoken words make up only a small part of communication. And while you may be already considering your response, you will be missing out on a large part of the message the speaker is trying to share with you.

Mindless communication is the opposite of mindful communication, which leads to mistrust, doubt, misunderstandings, and low morale. These will all damage your relationships, and hold you back from staying socially fit.

How to Improve Your Connections

There was a time when three generations would live together in one household, so any older adults were seldom alone. Through their contact with their children and interactions with their grandchildren's curious minds, they were never lonely, and the chance of mental decline was low. Today, older people may stay in one city and their children and grandchildren in another city or country. Now, older people are far more often surrounded by other people their age, who, like themselves, may be restricted in movement. And the chances for social interaction and mental stimulation are far less. If older people grow weak or need physical or psychological care or assistance, professionals take care of these needs. While I don't object to retirement complexes, this type of living can cause a disconnect from the rest of society.

How can you reconnect with the younger generations in your circle? Or keep these connections alive as every generation progresses through the various stages of life?

The following tips will help you close this gap:

- **Families that play together stay together.** Have fun with younger family members. Not only are you boosting your feel-good hormones, but you're also making magnificent memories while forming part of

your legacy. If play is limited, you can still have lots of fun.
- **Board and card games** are great ways to pass on new skills to your children and grandchildren and can lead to lots of laughter too. And just as important in these instances are the moments where trust is built, secrets are shared, and wisdom gets passed on.
- **Cooking is another fun activity**. A few weeks ago, I had dinner at a friend's house. While indulging in the most divine dessert, I asked for the recipe. She left to fetch her recipe book, a document that looked like a museum artifact as it belonged to her mother-in-law. It contained all the recipes she and her husband enjoyed making with her mother-in-law and they still continue to refer to for many different occasions.
- **It's now possible to talk to and see families who are living abroad**, thanks to the most astonishing technological advances. It can be done in real-time at a fraction of the cost it was only a decade or two ago. Once you become comfortable using technology, nothing is keeping you from checking in with family, even when they live far away in a completely different time zone.
- You can also benefit from **building relationships with others from different generations** that aren't related.
- **Get out of your home and step into the world**. Visit the park; make small talk at the grocery store; chat with your mailman, the UPS driver, or the cable guy. Immersing yourself in many seemingly insignificant interactions daily can help you remain socially fit.

- **Why not join a class to learn a new skill?** You can make friends in pottery classes, swim lessons, art classes, or any other interest you want to pursue.
- **Are you a fundraiser kind of gal or an avid gardener?** Whether you want to help save the planet, find the funds to keep the doors to your local community connection open, or help injured wildlife, you're likely to attract interest from like-minded people from all ages and walks of life.

THE IMPORTANCE OF PLAY

While we were young, we could spend hours playing. Then we grew older and forgot how to play. Play is not only a fun activity; more recently, research has revealed that play is essential for overall wellness.

The time you spend playing is essentially the time you put towards strengthening your mental health. Through play, you'll learn new skills, exercise your memory and creativity, and increase your focus. As play often requires physical activity, it's a way to remain fit and support your vitality. It also triggers the release of hormones that lift your spirit, and it's a great way to improve your outlook on life (Publisher, 2022). So start playing! Be happy and healthy and always surround yourself with people near and dear to you.

Play can include bowling, golf, tennis, badminton, pickleball or croquet, to name a few. If you're more of a creative spirit, you may enjoy creating art. dancing, acting, singing, or being a stand-up comedian may also interest you.

Another friend hosts regular social events at her home. These events are nothing fancy, and they're fun. She gathers friends for a fun casino night, Mexican fiesta, or card games. Sometimes, these events involve playing pool, competitive chess, poker night, or playing trivia games while sipping on some of the best wines.

Nature lovers may enjoy walking, hiking, photography, or flying kites. In comparison, the social butterfly might want to attend a beer festival, art show, carnival, or concert. As long as learning is fun, it can also constitute play. Learn how to write stories; knit; make pasta from scratch; make your own wine or beer; or get familiar with any other skill you want to learn. Animals can also add a lot of fun to your life. Are you a horse rider, dog walker, or cat lover? I dare you to find something near you, a place where you can go and have fun.

While all of these options I've listed above are wonderful ways to enjoy the benefits of play and overcome social gaps, it also helps eliminate the challenges of making new friends of any age. Let's face it, most of us reach an age where we're not as comfortable walking into a crowd of strangers and then walking away with many new friends. We can grow more reserved and stuck in our ways. However, all these activities create an excellent foundation to reach out and make new friends without stressing yourself.

DRESSING UP

What should you wear to these occasions? Having the perfect wardrobe may not be a challenge if you've been in the corporate world for most of your adult life. However, if you've been a stay-at-home mom, deciding on what to wear may be challenging, as you may want to look the part when you meet new friends. While at our age, we no longer dress to define our identity; we like to get dressed to express our individuality. So, what are some of the must-have items in your wardrobe?

Jeans are wonderfully versatile. Try finding a few cuts that compliment your body and have them in several shades. Jeans are lovely to pair with a blazer or a sweater. You can also stock up on different-colored shirts and fun-patterned blouses since they're great to wear underneath a blazer or on their own. When it comes to dresses, skirts, and anything else, always seek what compliments your body and leaves you feeling comfortable and confident. Confidence remains the best accessory regardless of what you wear at any age.

A FINAL WORD

- Age brings about a greater need to exercise your physical muscles and also your social skills. Letting both slide is easy, which can negatively impact your intentions of growing old successfully.
- You can increase your activity level in many ways, even if you're much older and think your time to be physically active has passed. Through exercising, you will have many health and wellness benefits. You will enjoy a greater sense of calm if you opt for mindful movement.

- Being socially active also becomes a matter of far greater importance when you get older.
- Modern society is structured in such a manner that you can easily be left out. So please use any of the ways explained in this chapter to remain socially active, have fun, stimulate your mind, and remain relevant.

STEP INTO A STRONGER IMMUNE SYSTEM

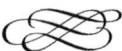

> *Laughter is timeless. Imagination has no age. And dreams are forever.*
>
> — WALT DISNEY

A widespread myth regarding aging and sleep assumes that the older you get, the less sleep you need. In reality, sleep remains as much a vital contributing factor to happy and healthy living when you're older as it is for a baby or a growing child. Even the National Sleep Foundation stipulates that adults can get away with less sleep until about the age of 60, but after that, the need for more sleep increases again; by the time you're 65, your body will need 7–8 hours of nightly sleep. Therefore, you need to be aware of changing factors impacting your sleep quality so you can effectively address these concerns, for even as a queen-ager, you still need your beauty sleep. And even greater importance is that your immune system needs to get enough sleep to ensure it remains in an optimal state, which will prevent an increased vulnerability to germs and diseases (Newsom, 2022).

UNDERSTANDING THE RELATIONSHIP BETWEEN SLEEP AND AGING

Lack of sleep is among the most prominent causes of various health concerns, especially after age 65. To successfully combat these concerns, you need to understand the relationship between sleep and aging (Newsom, 2022):

- Your circadian rhythm vastly impacts the length and quality of your sleep. This rhythm determines various functions of life, like hunger, alertness, and being sleepy. The hypothalamus in the brain is the area hosting your internal clock. As brain health deteriorates due to age, the clock becomes less effective in managing these cycles.
- Another contributing factor to the cycle being less accurate as we grow older is less exposure to sunlight. Changes can also be due to anxiety, depression, or certain medical conditions. The quality of life for older adults can also deteriorate over time, which can also impact the quality of sleep.

The results of these potential changes include:

- Noticeable earlier bedtimes and then waking up earlier in the morning.
- Waking up in the middle of the night and then struggling to fall asleep again. To wake up refreshed, you need to spend a certain amount of time in deep sleep. If you wake up often, your sleep cycle is fragmented, and you won't wake up rested.
- Many older adults nap during the day, and doing this, especially later in the day, makes it harder to fall asleep at night.
- You may struggle to adjust to new sleep schedules. Typical examples will be when you travel and find it much harder to recover from jet lag than when you were younger.

The Most Prominent Health Concerns Impacting Sleep

Several health concerns are more prevalent in older adults and keep you from getting the rest your body needs. Which of these concerns keeps you from getting the rest you need (Newsom, 2022)?

- Pain and discomfort—especially chronic pain or persistent discomfort—keeps many older adults awake at night. Lying still in one position can worsen your pain, causing you to wake up from constant body aches.
- Frequent urination during the night is another concern, since you must get up regularly to go to the bathroom.

- Feeling drowsy during the day is often due to medication or underlying health concerns.
- Sleep apnea—a condition where you wake up when you stop breathing—is far more common in older adults.
- Restless leg syndrome causes involuntary movement in your legs and feet, causing you to wake up.
- Insomnia is more common due to several other factors like stress and medication, resulting in the inability to fall asleep.
- REM disorder is another concern that causes you to move in your dreams and, as a result, wake up.

Tips to Help You Sleep Better

While the mere idea of not getting enough sleep is already exhausting, there's hope!

Identify Your Concern

Not all concerns keeping you from getting the rest you need are linked to age. By knowing which of the more common sleep concerns are related to aging, you can determine whether the challenges you face result from other problems or are merely symptoms of aging. Then you can start to address these concerns effectively. This is why it's crucial to identify your concerns accurately.

Suppose you experience any of the following symptoms along with sleep deprivation. Then your problems with sleep might require digging a little deeper. You may be actually battling a sleep disorder, which requires more attention:

- feeling constantly irritated
- struggling to concentrate
- being unable to fall back asleep
- not feeling refreshed when waking up
- needing alcohol or sleeping pills to fall asleep
- struggling to control your emotions
- falling asleep quickly when sitting down

Determine the Causes of Your Insomnia

You can only address a concern once you've identified it. So, what's keeping you awake at night or from falling asleep? Is it stress, feeling depressed, reliving past trauma, or even health concerns? The concerns can also be from menopause, side effects of medication, or inactivity during the day. Next time you lie awake, instead of desperately trying to fall asleep, shift your focus to determine what's keeping you awake.

Improve Your Sleep Habits

When you want to be healthy, you need to change your lifestyle and make healthier choices. The same is true for when you want to enjoy a better sleep. Here are some great choices when it comes to your sleep habits:

- Melatonin is linked to your circadian rhythm, and to ensure you have sufficient resources to maintain this rhythm, you can increase your melatonin by spending more time during the day exposed to sunlight. This will help improve your quality of sleep.

- Create a mental connection with your bedroom, by establishing it as a place where you're only intimate with your partner or to sleep. Suppose you're constantly going to work in your bedroom. In that case, your brain identifies it as a space where it needs to be alert, not naturally slowing down to fall asleep.
- You can also establish a sleep routine, which will help your brain wind down gradually until you have to go to sleep. Always going to bed at the same time every night will help too.
- While reading is a great way to help you fall asleep, you should avoid reading from devices with a backlight late at night, as the light waves of these devices keep your brain from shutting down.
- Have you tried stretching before bedtime or doing a few minutes of meditation? Having soothing rituals right before you go to bed also encourages quality sleep. I often write in my journal before going to bed, which has turned into a way to free my mind from the day's events.
- Try avoiding sleeping pills for as long as you can.
- When you take naps, ensure they are short and taken earlier in the day.

Improve Your Lifestyle to Improve Your Quality of Sleep

Lifestyle is undeniably linked to the quality of sleep you'll enjoy. And you'll enjoy better sleep by being more active, including healthier food options, and cutting down on sugary foods. While it can be hard to fall asleep while hungry, it's also not good to go to bed right after a heavy meal. Lying in bed with a full belly can lead to heartburn and feeling uncomfortable. It will also mean that your body is still actively busy with digestion and not entering a peaceful sleeping stage. Have caffeinated drinks earlier in the day, and try to avoid having drinks right before bedtime since this will result in getting up to urinate more often.

Once you increase your activity level during the day, you'll also notice an improvement in the quality of your sleep. Some exercise options that are light and work well in supporting a higher quality of sleep are taking regular brisk walks, cycling, or golfing. But why not add a fun social element to your exercises too? Try opting for something like dancing, socializing with friends, or playing fun games like bowling or pickleball.

Shed Some Stress

High levels of mental stress are among the greatest threats to having a high quality sleep pattern. Clear your mind by reading a good book, doing some stretching exercises, or include relaxation techniques in your bedtime routine—meditation will also help. If I struggle to fall asleep, I lay on my back with my hands on my belly and I shift my focus to the movement of my hands as I breathe in and out deeply. This will help minimize the influence of mental stress in your life too.

Getting enough sleep is vital to sustaining your overall wellness and ensuring longevity. While some factors impact your sleep without you having any control over them, you can still do many things to improve your situation, and those are the things you need to focus on.

HOW TO OPTIMIZE THE USE OF SUPPLEMENTS TO PROTECT YOUR IMMUNE DEFENSE SYSTEM

Besides getting enough sleep, you can also support your immune defense system by using supplements to build strength.

The ideal situation remains to get all the nutrition your body needs to stay fit, strong, and protected from disease through your diet. However, many factors can lead to a deficiency in this regard. As you age, turning to supplements to get the nutrition your body needs can become increasingly important.

Dietary supplements are available in several forms, like gels, tablets, capsules, liquids, or extracts, and they contain concentrated levels of certain nutrients. While you don't need a prescription to buy supplements, gathering information first to determine what your body needs and the best ways to answer this need is always suitable. Another point of interest is not all supplements are high quality. So don't settle for the most affordable options. Instead, seek out supplements with an excellent reputation for high quality ingredients.

While it will always be helpful to discuss dietary supplements you are taking or plan to include in your daily routine with your doctor first, the following will serve as a general guideline regarding what supplements can be beneficial at certain stages of aging:

- **In your 50s:** This is when it becomes increasingly important to take care of bone mass. Therefore, consider increasing your vitamin D and calcium intake. The two nutrients need to go together to be optimally effective. Nutrients that are important throughout your entire life but increasingly so after your 50s are omega-3, omega-6, and omega-9 fatty acids. These are found in oils and help reduce the odds of cholesterol concerns, support brain health, and play a vital role in managing blood sugar levels. Lastly, consider adding probiotics to your regimen, which cares for gut health. Your gut plays a central role in protecting your body from bacteria and ensuring efficient nutrient uptake.

- **In your 60s:** The likelihood of a vitamin-B deficiency rippling out to cause various health concerns like dementia can rapidly increase and best to avoid. So while you should continue with the supplements already mentioned, consider adding vitamin B and look into organic Ashwagandha or Lion's Mane for your cognitive health too.
- **In your 70s:** You should continue with B vitamins, vitamin D, calcium, omega-3-6-9, and probiotics. And since this is a stage when muscle mass can deteriorate, you should also consider increasing your protein intake.

Besides taking supplements, you can also include specific foods high in these nutrients.

Of course, dairy products remain an excellent source of calcium. Also consider having tuna and egg yolks in your diet to increase vitamin D. Salmon, flaxseed, and walnuts are great omega-3-6-9 fatty acids. At the same time, you can find probiotics in all fermented foods like yogurt, kefir, and sauerkraut. Dark chocolate is another excellent source of probiotics (Paturel, n.d.). Trout, clams, and hormone free, lean beef are all high in B vitamins, and you'll also be able to up your protein intake from beans, almonds, and chicken.

FIGHTING AGAINST FORGETFULNESS

Forgetfulness is one of the most frustrating aspects of aging. Still, even in this situation, you are not left entirely helpless, and you don't have to take a forgetful memory lying down. You can take several steps to prevent memory loss from impacting your life.

First, I want to highlight the immense difference between age-related memory loss and dementia. While the latter is a medical concern, age-related memory loss is a natural part of aging, happening to everyone. Yet, you can still take various measures to reduce its impact on your life. Before jumping right in, let's explore what this concern entails:

Age-related memory loss results from the hippocampus in the brain that is shrinking. This specific area in the brain is where you store your memories, and it merely starts to shrink due to age. While this deterioration occurs, your body is also slowing down in producing the hormones and proteins necessary to care for cell repair in this area. So, while deterioration begins to occur more rapidly, how your body would usually maintain such decline is also slowing down. As increased age often accompanies decreased activity, circulation slows down too, causing a reduced blood flow to the brain, further contributing to the concern.

These types of brain changes manifesting in your life are caused by the following results:

- You may find yourself struggling more often to find a specific word, as it remains stuck on the tip of your tongue.
- You might walk into a room and not recall why you went there.
- Being unable to remember where you've left things or placed them for safekeeping.

Increased Levels of Distraction

These are all symptoms of mere forgetfulness and not dementia. Between a positive diagnosis of dementia and forgetfulness, we find mild cognitive impairment (MCI). MCI has several more severe symptoms than mere concerns due to age. These symptoms include struggling to talk, thinking, or making severe judgment errors. MCI can also develop into Alzheimer's disease. In some cases, it can reach a plateau. In other cases, memory has returned to normal. Symptoms indicating that you might be dealing with the greater severity of MCI are when you often misplace things, forget the names of people you know, when you miss appointments regularly, or when it becomes harder to have a flowing conversation (Smith et al., 2022a).

When you experience these concerns more often, and it turns into everyday problems impacting your quality of life, it's important to schedule an appointment with your doctor to do all the necessary tests.

Lower Your Stress Levels to Improve Your Memory

One key contributing factor to memory loss is persistent high stress levels. I'm referring specifically to high levels of cortisol. *Cortisol* is designed to be a lifesaver. Our ancestors could survive through this stress hormone when they had to protect themselves against predators. We no longer live in an environment where our lives are regularly threatened. However, the hormone causing the fight-or-flight response is still primarily at play, making us stressed and on high alert. Yet, the problem is while our bodies are designed to react well to a surge of cortisol, we don't do so well when there's prolonged exposure to this stress hormone.

Cortisol impacts several areas of the brain, and the part most relevant to memory loss is the deterioration it causes to the *prefrontal cortex*. This specific brain area is essential for short-term memory. When it deteriorates, you'll struggle to remember where your keys are placed or why you came into the kitchen.

So, by reducing your stress levels today, you can preserve your memory for tomorrow.

Get enough sleep, exercise, maintain healthy relationships, and be kind to yourself. Other proven ways to reduce stress is caring for a pet, being more spiritual, eating healthy, taking supplements, identifying stressful thoughts when you have them, and often laughing because having fun is a great way to drop your stress levels too.

HOW IMPORTANT IS HUMOR?

Who doesn't like a great laugh? The problem with laughing is that we don't do it often enough. As you grow older, you should allow more space in your life for humor since laughing is one of the best ways to effortlessly drop your stress levels and protect your memory from the impact of cortisol. Just think back to the last time you had a great laugh. You know, one of those where your belly or face ached afterward. How did it make you feel? Did it change your mood? Of course it did! Laughter is a proven way to reduce stress and make you feel so much better. These are not mere assumptions about laughter but actually proven facts. Clinical studies show that laughter plays a significant role in improving memory, learning disabilities, short-term memory, and it speeds up the process of recalling information. Researchers consider laughter a workout for the brain ("The Benefits of Humor," 2017).

There are many jokes about aging and how it's no laughing matter. Suppose you still fail to see how including humor and having a regular laugh can improve your overall mental health. In that case, the joke is on you! It's not nearly as funny as the ones that could've done wonders to preserve your memory. So, for the love of Pete, John, Adam or whoever else you can think of, have a good laugh!

A FINAL WORD

- As you grow older, you become increasingly vulnerable in two specific areas of your being: immune defense and memory.
- There are several contributing factors causing a decline in these areas. Still, you're not a helpless bystander, having to merely watch how your life deteriorates. In both instances, there are several steps you can take to improve your situation.
- Getting enough sleep is at the heart of protecting your immune system.
- There are several reasons why you may struggle to sleep as well as you used to, and here I've included several steps you can take to improve your quality of sleep.
- By opting for supplements, you can further strengthen your body's ability to protect itself.
- It's important to distinguish between age-related memory loss and dementia.
- We all suffer a memory decline because certain parts of the brain deteriorates as we age.
- Know the symptoms you are experiencing and keep track of any changes to your situation.
- MCI is more severe than age-related memory loss. While it can reach a plateau and even be reversed, it can also lead to Alzheimer's disease. So make sure you know when to get a medical assessment.

- You can also protect your memory and slow aging by reducing stress levels. The best and easiest way to do this is to laugh and to laugh often.

Now that I've shared all the tips and solutions I've learned on my journey and from my years of researching the topic of how to age successfully, I want us to move on to how you can step into your power and reclaim control of your life so that your future and growing older gracefully is something you will look forward to.

STEP INTO YOUR POWER!

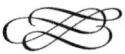

> *Beautiful young people are accidents of nature, but beautiful old people are works of art.*
>
> — ELEANOR ROOSEVELT

The only thing we can ever truly be sure of is change. For some, this is a fear-provoking matter. Others look forward to it with anticipation.

CHANGE IS AN INEVITABLE PART OF LIFE

When you put your hand into a flowing river, you'll never be able to touch the same water twice. This serves as an anecdote that time is always passing and changing, and you'll never be able to relive a specific moment again. However, somewhere between hearing and understanding these stories' lessons and applying them to our lives, something gets lost. We gain wisdom but fail to apply it.

By this stage of the book, you know that every day, hour, minute, and even second that goes by is time that you'll never regain, never be able to relive. Yet, it can be challenging to remain present in the moment while it's easy to drift off on a cloud of worries about the future or get lost in a thick fog of regret over mistakes in the past.

I want to remind you that change is inevitably part of life. The moment you have now, you'll never have again. The person you are at this exact moment, you'll never be again. The idea of passing the time away is something that should increase our appreciation for every moment we have. Yet, so many lose focus of the present moment as they are filled with dread or even fear while watching their time run out.

Use the realization that change is constantly happening as a reminder and encouragement to emphasize the importance of being more mindful and cultivate greater awareness of your present experiences. Employ mindfulness and meditation to make awareness a habit. This awareness of the present is an excellent foundation to set you on the right track to claim your power.

CULTIVATE A POSITIVE MINDSET

From this foundation, sprouts positivity. A positive mindset is more than merely something that makes your life pleasant. Positivity is also a feature that supports successful aging.

Research indicates that a positive approach to life contributes to faster healing and recovery and slows down aging as it's directly linked to lower blood pressure, supporting heart health (Severson, 2012).

A positive attitude also radiates from any queen-ager and helps support her quest to implement healthy habits. When I make such a statement, I'm not referring to a fickle and shallow pretentiousness that all is dandy. I'm referring to a much deeper experience rooted in the knowledge that, at times, things won't look as rosy as you would like them to be. Still, you remain confident in your ability to replace negative—and often unfounded—thoughts with positive ones. It's a positivity secured by the certainty that you have strong bonds that have been established with people you can count on when the going gets tough.

This positivity continues to spark a curiosity to know more, learn more, and become more. Such a positive approach to life will lead you towards enjoying your golden years because you'll do what is necessary to stay relevant by upskilling yourself with technological advancements and planning ahead to ensure not a day goes by without being significant in some regard. It's the kind of positive approach to life that doesn't matter how many times you fall but how many times you get up to continue upwards and onwards so you can enjoy your life.

SPIRITUALITY AND AGING

Maybe you've always been spiritual or haven't cared about spirituality that much throughout your entire life. Yet, now is a great time to explore spirituality as it can gather greater interest as we age and is linked with overall wellness in older adults. Studies even indicate that the comfort found in spirituality can increase longevity (Elder Care Alliance, 2017).

The increased importance of spirituality as we age is connected to spirituality being a coping mechanism for many. Old age brings about many concerns, especially ones linked to your health. And, you can find comfort in the deeper connections in spiritual practice; that way, you can use it as a coping mechanism. Many older adults also rely upon spiritual practice to expand their social connections and find comfort in others sharing the same values and beliefs.

Pursuing spiritual wellness is a way to secure a positive approach to life despite facing hardship. Spiritual wellness asks that you look beyond your limitations, which may decline with time, so you can find meaning and purpose in your life. Having a purpose and gaining confirmation that none of the challenges and adversities you've faced and are still facing are meaningless, contributes to an overall positive approach to life (Mary's Woods, n.d.).

HOW TO PURSUE SPIRITUAL WELLNESS

I urge you to pursue spiritual wellness, but I don't want you to confuse it as a call to increase religiousness against your will. Religion is only one part of spirituality, and you can enjoy spiritual wellness in many ways without becoming devoted to any specific religion.

Meditation, being more creative, and spending time in nature are all significant steps toward spiritual wellness. Spending time in nature is an excellent way to reduce your stress level, and it's where you'll feel a stronger connection with the entire universe. Take a moment and become aware of your connection with the universe and how you're part of something much larger than what your life may reflect.

There are several ways you can use spiritual activities to make this connection. By strengthening your relationship with yourself through meditation or yoga, finding a purpose in life through volunteering, or even getting involved in a meaningful project. Helping others and expressing gratitude and appreciation towards them can help you connect with others. You can also connect to the world more effectively by spending time in nature, gardening, walking, or—even if your mobility is restricted—gathering plants in your living space. Being surrounded by nature encourages us to make the most of our life and inspires us to be creative. Spiritual connections bring us closer to the larger universe, others, and ourselves. It gives purpose and meaning and adds value to life, leaving you feeling energized and happy.

MENTORING YOUNGER GENERATIONS

You've walked the walk, and now you're more than capable of talking the talk. In short, the older you get, the more experience you have. Why not pass your wisdom on to the younger generations? Share the knowledge with those eager to learn. While the world may be an ever-changing place, there are always some principles that remain valid all the time. Therefore the experience you have doesn't age. You place yourself in a respected position by sharing your stories with younger generations. It's a way to increase your confidence and find a new purpose in life.

Several research studies are revealing the importance of intergenerational mentoring. Through this type of contact, you remain valid in a society where younger generations are now the leaders. It serves as a way to overcome the generation gap and the isolation you may experience. However, it's more than just today's leaders relying on older generations' guidance. Modern society is a place with many youngsters eager to find a mentor they can turn to for advice and guidance, someone who can share the ropes of adulthood and how to successfully overcome some of the obstacles they're facing. Youngsters with an adult mentor generally do better academically, are better prepared for adulthood and are more positively inclined toward the future (Bosak, n.d.). Previously, we also discussed the many benefits older adults reap from such a relationship. These are benefits that include being more positive and purpose-driven.

What does effective mentoring look like? Before taking on such a venture, you must be clear about your intentions and what you want to gain from it. You also have to know what you're willing to invest in such a relationship, as mentoring requires a lot of time, and you must be committed to the relationship. Mentors who are authentic in their approach; willing to give the relationship time until a trusting bond has developed; sensitive towards the mentee's boundaries, past experiences, and other differences; and consistent in this position as a role model, do best in this position. You also have to make your expectations of your mentee known from the start. Ultimately, this is a mutually beneficial relationship rooted in mutual respect.

It's also a relationship that will experience bumps and challenges along the way, so prepare yourself for obstacles and even resistance from your mentee from time to time. Remember that you're the role model, not a parent or caregiver. The mentee can rely on you for advice, but you're not responsible for them to make the choices and complete the actions that will benefit them.

ENGAGE IN MEANINGFUL SOCIALIZATION

We've established by now that the older you get, the more valuable it is to have meaningful relationships. It's a way to develop yourself, expand your horizons by allowing diversity to enter your world, and allows you to gain access to a support network. Also, these relationships can propel you forward as they add meaning to your present and future life.

Older adults who connect to social networks and have access to deep and meaningful relationships enjoy greater longevity. The increased life expectancy they enjoy is the result of greater physical and mental health, so they're less likely to deal with depression, and they enjoy a better quality of life in general (*Importance of Socialization*, 2019).

Suppose you're in a position where you struggle with mobility and are dependent on others to move around. You may feel like you're being cut off from the world and can no longer socialize. Perhaps you don't feel as mentally sharp anymore and might be anxious about social settings out of fear you'll embarrass yourself. There are ways you can overcome these obstacles too. If you're socializing with others of a similar age as yourself, they're likely to not notice if you struggle and are even more likely to understand what you're going through. When the crowd you're in is younger, you'll soon find they'll appreciate your presence more. While you may feel insecure, younger generations look up to you with the greatest respect, appreciation, and understanding. It all depends on how willing you are to engage with others.

Here are some ways you can reduce stress linked to socializing with others:

- Start by joining groups where the attention will only be on you some of the time, like joining a community group or book club.
- You can also start small and invite a friend or relative to have tea or coffee at your home. I organize live Zoom get-togethers with my friends each month, allowing us to connect and share what's been happening in our lives since most of us live in different cities. It's a great way to share recipes, financial wisdom, and what's new in each of our lives.
- Some find it easier to socialize when there's a specific purpose linked to the interaction, and it's not merely

about making small talk initially. Then, it will help to volunteer, join a community project, help kids with homework, or even babysit if you are physically fit to take on such a responsibility. Even chatting with others as you go through your daily activities can be a form of casual social interaction, leaving you feeling great. Are you ready to make minor changes in your life as a first step to start building deep and meaningful bonds?

What are the risks linked to a lack of social connection? Regardless of how introverted you are, people are social beings, and we need some social activity to flourish. Some consequences of limiting your interactions with others include lowered self-esteem and exposure to being at high risk for specific medical concerns like cancer, depression, and mental health conditions (*Importance of Socialization*, 2019). It also leads to losing confidence in your ability to cope with others or even to show compassion. Engaging in social activity is one of the vital steps to propel yourself forward to a future that leaves you feeling motivated and filled with anticipation over all the possibilities it holds.

LET'S GET PRACTICAL

Are you excited about change or trapped in the shadows of fear of what the unknown holds? As aging—heck, life in general—is synonymous with change, I want you to immerse yourself in the following exercise.

1. Pick a window in your home with a view of outside activity. Stand firm with both feet securely on the ground, and start to feel the pressure of your weight on the soles of your feet and how gravity pulls you to the floor. Become aware that even though you're standing still, there's still movement. Earth is still spinning on its axis, and life continues as usual. Then, expand your focus. First, explore the things or people closest to you and then move further away, taking in every little detail. Can you see how change is happening? Maybe you see people moving in the street, a lady jogging, a moving van unloading furniture for new neighbors, or the postal worker doing deliveries. If your view is mostly on a natural scene, see if any birds or bugs fly about or if the wind gently pushes the tree leaves around. Do you notice that the entire world is constantly changing? And even though you are standing still, is there constant movement and change all around you?
2. Now, shift your focus toward yourself. What are the changes you observe in your body? What sensations are you feeling? Did your breathing change, or your heart rate slow down? You may feel the tension building somewhere in your body, or some muscles may feel more relaxed.
3. Take a moment to think about how everything in the world changes, inside and outside your body. Accept these changes, as change indicates progress and, in fact, a sign of life. Immerse yourself for a moment and appreciate the much bigger, changing world you're part of before turning towards your journal.

4. In your journal, reflect on the emotions you've experienced during the exercise. Did you feel fear, concern, excitement, or an increased sense of peace with the changes you witnessed? Did the fact that you experienced change internally while witnessing it outside make you feel more connected with your environment? As if you truly belong where you are? Does this feeling increase your confidence that you're in a secure space and in an excellent position to propel yourself toward your future?

A FINAL WORD

- How you experience growing older will be exactly how you perceive it. If you're dreading it, you're increasing the odds that it will be a time you'll feel depressed, sick, exhausted, and as if your life has no meaning or purpose.
- However, you can also perceive getting older as a time to look forward to, when you'll enjoy peace, joy, and positivity, and feel meaningful.
- Throughout this book, I've shared tips that worked for me to help change my perspective on getting older.
- These changes resulted in me enjoying a meaningful life. They allow me to enjoy my older adult years while having a purpose, being connected, and feeling happy and excited.
- Getting older is a substantial part of anyone's life, and it's truly a blessing when you have a long life.

- How you live these golden years is up to you. I hope you take the knowledge I've shared to step into your power, a position where your life can be more meaningful than what you may have thought in your younger years.

CONCLUSION

Throughout our lives, we gather stories and snippets of wisdom. Sometimes we forget them as soon as we hear them, only to show up again when relevant. Other stories make a lasting impression and are crucial in shaping our lives.

One such story that remains very relevant to me is the one about the two sons of an alcoholic dad. The one son became an alcoholic just like his father, and he would state that he was drinking because he saw that was what his father did. The other son didn't touch alcohol and said he did this because he saw what his father did (Krueger & Foster, 2008).

The lesson: Regardless of what your life looked like until now, you can change it today. Even if your life up until this point was characterized by unhealthy eating habits; lack of exercise; perceiving people and your relationships as a mere means to an end; or whatever you've been up to, you still have the choice to make that change today. The freedom to use all the steps and exercises I've provided remains yours. It was a choice I'm so grateful I made 10 years ago and one I hope you will be thankful to make today!

I've covered what taking stock of your life means and how the lessons you learn by taking a step back can improve your future. The level of satisfaction you'll enjoy from any journey is influenced mainly by the state of your vehicle. For this journey, your body is your vehicle. And we've explored physical health and how to care for your mental and emotional well-being.

Some people know exactly who they are when they are kids, while others age a bit more to find their authentic selves. It doesn't matter how long you've been seeking your authentic self. What matters is that you find it so you can live with purpose and motivation. Once you do, it becomes so much easier to love yourself, to love others, and to love your life. It's when you gain the confidence and the desire to reach out to others and to strengthen your bonds, a mutually beneficial venture adding so much value to your life, enabling you to enjoy the highest quality of life, a life of contentment and one in which you can sustain a positive outlook, even in the face of adversity.

I want you to enjoy your golden years. I want you to live a life of joy, fulfillment, and lasting mental, physical, and emotional wellness. I want you to age successfully, and I hope this book inspires and motivates you to pursue this goal.

Have you gained any insights you hoped for when you started this journey? Then please share your experience by leaving a positive review on Amazon, encouraging other women to learn how they can step into their powers too!

With the following words of Walter D. Wintle, I want to send you off on your journey of successful aging as you step more into your power each and every day! (Wintle, 1905):

> *"If you think you are beaten, you are*
> *If you think you dare not, you don't*
> *If you like to win, but you think you can't*
> *It is almost certain you won't.*
>
> *If you think you'll lose, you're lost*
> *For out of the world we find,*
> *Success begins with a person's will-*
> *It's all in the state of mind.*
>
> *If you think you are outclassed, you are,*
> *You've got to think high to rise.*
> *You've got to be sure of yourself before*
> *You can ever win a prize.*
>
> *Life's battles don't always go*
> *to the strongest or fastest*
> *But sooner or later the one who wins*
> *Is the one who thinks they can!"*

THE FINAL STEP

As you embrace your authentic self and step into the future with positivity and vitality, you put yourself in the perfect position to help other women to do the same… and that's as easy as writing a review.

Simply by sharing your honest opinion of this book on Amazon, you'll show other readers where they can find the same inspiration and guidance that brought you to this page.

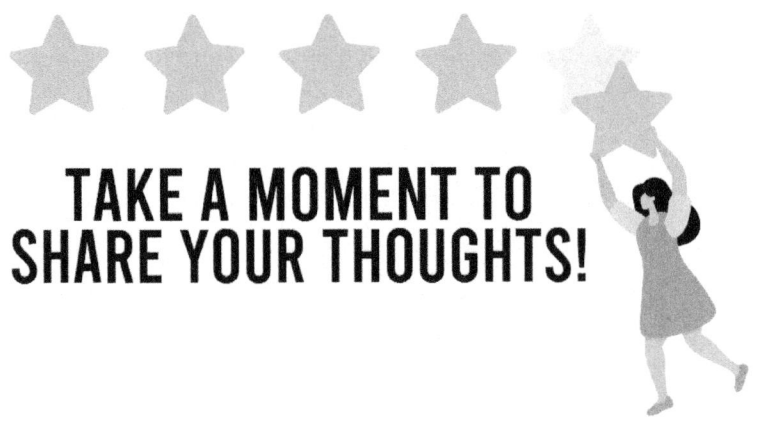

Thank you so much for your support. Step forward into your best life knowing you've helped someone else to do the same.

REFERENCES

Adams, K. B. (2012, August 6). *Banishing mid-life regret*. Psychology Today. https://www.psychologytoday.com/intl/blog/mid-life-what-crisis/201208/banishing-mid-life-regret

Authentic relationships—Do you have a genuine connection?. (2021, November 19). Harley Therapy Counseling Blog. https://www.harleytherapy.co.uk/counselling/authentic-relationships.htm

The benefits of humor as we age. (n.d.). FirstLight Home Care. https://www.firstlighthomecare.com/blog/the-benefits-of-humor-as-we-age/

Bertin, M. (2017, September 25). *A 5-minute mindful breathing practice to restore your attention. Mindful*. https://www.mindful.org/5-minute-mindful-breathing-practice-restore-attention/

Bosak, S. V. (n.d.). *Effective mentoring*. Legacy Project. https://www.legacyproject.org/guides/mentors.html

Bowie, D. (n.d.). *Aging is an extraordinary process whereby you become the person you always should have been* [Quote]. Quotefancy. https://quotefancy.com/quote/2023132/David-Bowie-Aging-is-an-extraordinary-process-whereby-you-become-the-person-you-always

Breeding, B. (2018, July 23). *Positive aging: Changing your mindset about growing older*. myLiftSite. https://mylifesite.net/blog/post/positive-aging-changing-mindset-growing-older/

Burn, G. (n.d.). *You can't help getting older, but you don't have to get old* [Quote]. BrainyQuote. https://www.brainyquote.com/quotes/george_burns_103932

Capetta, A., & Muenter, O. (2022, July 14). *17 signs you're having a midlife crisis*. Woman's Day. https://www.womansday.com/health-fitness/wellness/g2966/signs-of-midlife-crisis-in-a-woman/

Caraballo, M. (n.d.). *Forgiving yourself and moving forward | The best new year gift*. Cheers to Chapter Two. https://cheers2chapter2.com/forgiving-yourself-and-moving-forward-the-best-new-year-gift

Catherine, L. (2019, July 23). *Authentic relationships are important—see the good in connection* Choose to See Good. https://choosetoseegood.com/authentic-relationships-are-important-see-the-good-in-connection/

Chilangwa, P. A. (2021). *Mindfulness practices for women's midlife transition* [Master's Thesis, Lesley University]. Institutional Repositories.

Davidson, K. (2020, February 5). *9 healthy foods to lift your mood.* Healthline. https://www.healthline.com/nutrition/mood-food

Davidson, K. (2021, June 14). *11 natural ways to lower your cortisol levels.* Healthline. https://www.healthline.com/nutrition/ways-to-lower-cortisol

Degges-White, S. (2014, April 1). *Midlife: Ripe, juicy, authentic relationships.* Psychology Today. https://www.psychologytoday.com/us/blog/lifetime-connections/201404/midlife-ripe-juicy-authentic-relationships

Disney, W. (n.d.). *Laughter is timeless, imagination has no age, dreams are forever* [Quote]. Quotefancy. https://quotefancy.com/quote/757122/Walt-Disney-Laughter-is-timeless-imagination-has-no-age-dreams-are-forever

Elder Care Alliance. (2017, January 17). *Seniors and spirituality: Health benefits of faith.* https://eldercarealliance.org/blog/seniors-and-spirituality-health-benefits-of-faith/

Friedan, B. (n.d.). *Aging is not lost youth but a new stage of opportunity and strength* [Quote]. BrainyQuote. https://www.brainyquote.com/quotes/betty_friedan_383994

Gillam, D. (n.d.). *Aging is a laughing matter.* Age Wise King County. https://www.agewisekingcounty.org/ill_pubs_articles/aging-laughing-matter/

The Greenfields Continuing Care Community. (n.d.). *5 benefits of exercise for seniors and aging adults.* https://thegreenfields.org/5-benefits-exercise-seniors-aging-adults/

Roosevelt, E. (n.d.). *Beautiful young people are accidents of nature, but beautiful old people are works of art* [Quote]. Quotefancy. https://quotefancy.com/quote/799782/Eleanor-Roosevelt-Beautiful-young-people-are-accidents-of-nature-but-beautiful-old-people

Harrogate. (n.d.). *Find your purpose by exploring spirituality as you grow older.* https://www.harrogatelifecare.org/news/exploring-your-spiritual-side/

Harvard Pilgrim Health Care. (n.d.). *Science of food and aging.* https://www.harvardpilgrim.org/hapiguide/the-science-of-food-and-aging/

Harvard University. (2017, May 1). *What does it take to be a super-ager?* https://www.health.harvard.edu/healthy-aging/what-does-it-take-to-be-a-super-ager

Haslam, N. (2019, October 14). *Why the "midlife crisis" is a myth.* CNN. https://edition.cnn.com/2019/10/14/health/midlife-crisis-the-conversation-wellness/index.html

Healthy aging: How volunteering helps. (n.d.). Parentgiving. https://www.parentgiving.com/elder-care/healthy-aging-how-volunteering-helps/

Hepburn, A. (n.d.). And the beauty of a woman, with passing years only grows [Quote]! Goodreads. https://www.goodreads.com/quotes/133783-and-the-beauty-of-a-woman-with-passing-years-only

Hogan, L. (2021, August 25). *How to be more empathetic.* WebMD. https://www.webmd.com/balance/features/how-to-be-more-empathetic

How helping others benefits you. (n.d.). New Jersey City University. https://www.njcu.edu/student-life/campus-services-resources/counseling-center/additional-resources/articles/how-helping-others-benefits-you

Importance of socialization as we age. (2019, August 5). Avista Senior Living. https://avistaseniorliving.com/the-importance-of-socialization-as-we-age/

Improving connections among different generations. (n.d.). Sage Minder. https://www.sageminder.com/Caregiving/Relationships/ConnectingGenerations.aspx

Inge, C. (n.d.). *How to define your personal core values.* Human Design With Christie Inge. https://christieinge.com/personal-core-values/

Intermountain Health Care. (2019, March 8). *7 ways kindness improves your health.* https://intermountainhealthcare.org/blogs/topics/live-well/2019/03/7-ways-kindness-improves-your-health/

Janac, S. (2018, October 8). *Self care for midlife women | TBB linkup.* The Queen in Between. https://www.thequeeninbetween.com/self-care-for-midlife-women-tbb-linkup/

Kets de Vries, M. F. R. (2016, December 21). Make peace with your unlived life. *Harvard Business Review.* https://hbr.org/2016/12/make-peace-with-your-unlived-life

Krueger, G., & Foster, M. -L. (2008, June 11). *A story about 1 father and his 2 sons with 3 lessons for all of us.* Bigg Success. https://biggsuccess.com/2008/06/11/1-father-2-sons-3-lessons-for-all-of-us/

Lam, M., & Lam, D. (n.d.). *Sugar and aging: Implications to healthy living.* Dr. Lam Coaching. https://www.drlamcoaching.com/blog/sugar-and-aging/

Lawson, K. (n.d.). *How do thoughts and emotions affect health?* University of Minnesota. https://www.takingcharge.csh.umn.edu/how-do-thoughts-and-emotions-affect-health

Lee, R. (n.d.). *Living an authentic life by finding your true self.* Midlifing It. https://midlifingit.com/living-an-authentic-life-by-finding-your-true-self/

Life Begins At. (2017, September 20). *How to overcome the invisible woman phenomenon*. Life Begins At Magazine. https://www.lifebeginsat.com.au/overcome-invisible-woman-phenomenon/

Lisa. (n.d.). *5 reasons to learn 5 new things in midlife*. Midlife Pursuits. https://midlifepursuits.com/5-reasons-to-learn-5-new-things-in-midlife/

MacArthur, D. (n.d.). *Years may wrinkle the skin, but to give up interest wrinkles the soul. You are as young as your faith, as old as your doubt; as young as your self-confidence, as old as your fear; as young as your hope as old as your despair. In the central place of every heart there is a recording chamber. So long as it receives messages of beauty, hope, cheer and courage, so long are you young. When your heart is covered with the snows of pessimism and the ice of cynicism, then, and then only, are you grown old. And then, indeed as the ballad says, you just fade away* [Quote]. Goodreads. https://www.goodreads.com/quotes/413531-years-may-wrinkle-the-skin-but-to-give-up-interest

Mary's Woods. (n.d.). *Importance of spirituality as we age*. https://maryswoods.org/blog/spirituality-seniors/

Mattson, A., & Radley, J. (2014, June 17). *Stress hormone linked to short-term memory loss as we age*. University of Iowa. https://now.uiowa.edu/2014/06/stress-hormone-linked-short-term-memory-loss-we-age

Mawri, S. (2022, August 3). *Beware high levels of cortisol, the stress hormone*. Premier Health. https://www.premierhealth.com/your-health/articles/women-wisdom-wellness-/beware-high-levels-of-cortisol-the-stress-hormone

Meyer, J. (2017, October 27). *You are more than your mistakes*. Thought Catalog. https://thoughtcatalog.com/jillian-meyer/2017/10/you-are-more-than-your-mistakes/

Mindfulness for older adults (infographic). (n.d.). Be Independent HomeCare. https://www.beindependenthomecare.ie/mindfulness-for-older-adults/

Moulds, C. (n.d.). *7 ways for midlife women to overcome self-doubt*. Cara Moulds. https://www.caramoulds.com/7-ways-for-midlife-women-to-overcome-self-doubt/

Nall, R. (2018, May 29). *Life review therapy*. Healthline. https://www.healthline.com/health/life-review-therapy

National Institutes of Health. (2015, November). *Positive emotions and your health: Developing a brighter outlook*. U.S. Department of Health and Human

Services. https://newsinhealth.nih.gov/2015/08/positive-emotions-your-health

National Institute on Aging. (n.d.). *10 myths about aging*. U.S. Department of Health and Human Services, National Institutes of Health. https://www.nia.nih.gov/health/10-myths-about-aging

National Institute on Aging. (2021, April 23). *Dietary supplements for older adults*. U.S. Department of Health and Human Services, National Institutes of Health. https://www.nia.nih.gov/health/dietary-supplements-older-adults

Newsom, R. (2022, March 18). *Aging and sleep*. Sleep Foundation. https://www.sleepfoundation.org/aging-and-sleep

Picasso, P. (n.d.). *It takes a long time to become young* [Quote]. BrainyQuote. https://www.brainyquote.com/quotes/pablo_picasso_103938

Paturel, A. (n.d.). *Supplements to take in your 50s, 60s and 70s*. AARP. https://www.aarp.org/health/drugs-supplements/info-2015/must-have-supplements.html

Phillips, M. L. (2011, April). *The mind at midlife*. American Psychological Association. https://www.apa.org/monitor/2011/04/mind-midlife

Promises Behavioral Health. (2012, June 27) *Life review therapy helps alleviate depression in the elderly*. https://www.promises.com/addiction-blog/life-review-therapy/

Providence Senior Health Team. (2020, November 22). *Positive pursuit of a new purpose after midlife*. Providence. https://blog.providence.org/blog-2/the-positive-pursuit-of-a-new-purpose-after-midlife

Publisher. (2022, April 22). *Fun activities for seniors: Over 100 ways to play*. GreatSeniorLiving. https://www.greatseniorliving.com/articles/fun-activities-for-seniors

Pulsifer, C., & Gillison, B. (n.d.). 57 quotes about helping others. Inspirational Words of Wisdom. https://www.wow4u.com/helping/

Ridsdel, J. (2021, April 1). *10 common negative thinking patterns and 5 steps for change*. The Family Centre. https://www.familycentre.org/news/post/10-common-negative-thinking-patterns-and-5-steps-for-change

Robinson, L., & Segal, J. (2023, January 2). *Eating well as you age*. Help Guide. https://www.helpguide.org/articles/healthy-eating/eating-well-as-you-age.htm

Rock, L. (2018, May 5). *Life gets better after 50: Why age tends to work in favour of happiness*. The Guardian. https://www.theguardian.com/lifeandstyle/2018/may/05/happiness-curve-life-gets-better-after-50-jonathan-rauch

Rosales, A. (2018, May 12). *Mindfulness meditation at midlife: What, why and how*. Jubilant Age. https://jubilantage.com/mindfulness-meditation-at-midlife-what-why-and-how/

Roosevelt, T. (n.d.). *It is not the critic who counts; not the man who points out how the strong man stumbles, or where the doer of deeds could have done them better. The credit belongs to the man who is actually in the arena, whose face is marred by dust and sweat and blood; who strives valiantly; who errs, who comes short again and again, because there is no effort without error and shortcoming; but who does actually strive to do the deeds; who knows great enthusiasms, the great devotions; who spends himself in a worthy cause; who at the best knows in the end the triumph of high achievement, and who at the worst, if he fails, at least fails while daring greatly, so that his place shall never be with those cold and timid souls who neither know victory nor defeat* [Quote]. Goodreads. https://www.goodreads.com/quotes/7-it-is-not-the-critic-who-counts-not-the-man

Sage Neuroscience Center. (2021, November 19). *Breaking the cycle: Negative thought patterns*. https://sageclinic.org/blog/negative-thoughts-depression/

Schlafman, S. (2018, December 24). *How to conduct an annual life review that will catapult you into the new year*. Medium. https://schlaf.medium.com/how-to-conduct-an-annual-life-review-that-will-catapult-you-into-the-new-year-d5aaffebac1f

7 best exercises for seniors (and a few to avoid!). (n.d.). Senior Lifestyle. https://www.seniorlifestyle.com/resources/blog/7-best-exercises-for-seniors-and-a-few-to-avoid/

Severson, A. (2012, November 20). *Positive thinking leads to better health in the elderly*. Healthline. https://www.healthline.com/health-news/positive-attitudes-help-seniors-recover-from-disability-112012

Shuckburgh, L. (2021, May 9). *Self-doubt*. Marvellous Midlife. https://www.marvellousmidlife.co.uk/blog/self-doubt

Siegle, S. (2020, May 29). *The art of kindness*. Mayo Clinic Heath System. https://www.mayoclinichealthsystem.org/hometown-health/speaking-of-health/the-art-of-kindness

Sirois, M. (n.d.). *How to apply positive psychology to the midlife journey*. Wholebeing Institute. https://wholebeinginstitute.com/positive-psychology-midlife-journey/

Smith, M., Robinson, L., & Segal, R. (2022a, December 5). *Age-related memory loss*. Help Guide. https://www.helpguide.org/articles/alzheimers-dementia-aging/age-related-memory-loss.htm

Smith, M., Robinson, L., & Segal, R. (2022b, December 5). *Sleep tips for older adults*. HelpGuide. https://www.helpguide.org/articles/sleep/how-to-sleep-well-as-you-age.htm

Sohn, L. (2019, July 3). *What do 90-somethings regret most? Here's what I learned about how to live a happy, regret-free life*. CNBC. https://www.cnbc.com/2019/07/03/advice-from-90-year-olds-how-to-live-a-long-happy-and-regret-free-life.html

Stelter, G. (2022, November 28). *How seniors can improve balance and stability with tai chi*. Healthline. https://www.healthline.com/health/senior-health/ta-chi

Stibich, M. (2020, February 4). *Embrace aging with positive thinking*. Verywell Mind. https://www.verywellmind.com/positive-thinking-and-aging-2224134

Stibich, M. (2022, September 24). *10 best brain games to keep your mind sharp*. Verywell Mind. https://www.verywellmind.com/top-websites-and-games-for-brain-exercise-2224140

Strenger, C., & Ruttenberg, A. (2008, February). The existential necessity of midlife change. *Harvard Business Review*. https://hbr.org/2008/02/the-existential-necessity-of-midlife-change

Success over 50: Top 10 career success stories. (2021, July 8). Careline365. https://www.careline.co.uk/success-top-10-late-bloomers/

Suttie, J. (2018, March 8). *How to find your purpose in midlife*. University of California, Berkely, Greater Good Science Center. https://greatergood.berkeley.edu/article/item/how_to_find_your_purpose_in_midlife

Teng, J. (n.d.). *Learn from the mistakes of others*. Midlife Magazine. https://livxtra.net/learn-from-the-mistakes-of-others/

Willsey, P. S. (2021, August 24). *Creating authentic connections*. Psychology Today. https://www.psychologytoday.com/us/blog/packing-success/202108/creating-authentic-connections

Wintle, W. D. (1905). *Thinking*. All Poetry. https://allpoetry.com/poem/8624439-Thinking-by-Walter-D-Wintle

Printed in Great Britain
by Amazon